Cochlear Implants: New Perspectives

Advances in Oto-Rhino-Laryngology

Vol. 48

Series Editor
C.R. Pfaltz, Basel

KARGER

Basel · Freiburg · Paris · London · New York · New Delhi · Bangkok · Singapore · Tokyo · Sydney

International Symposium, Toulouse, June 2–3, 1992

Cochlear Implants: New Perspectives

Volume Editors
B. Fraysse, O. Deguine, Toulouse

Volume Co-Editors
N. Cochard, Toulouse; *R. Dauman,* Bordeaux; *A. Uziel,* Toulouse

89 figures and 41 tables, 1993

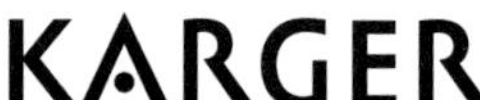

Basel · Freiburg · Paris · London · New York · New Delhi · Bangkok · Singapore · Tokyo · Sydney

Advances in Oto-Rhino-Laryngology

Library of Congress Cataloging-in-Publication Data
Cochlear implants: new perspectives: international symposium, Toulouse, June 2–3, 1992/ volume editors, B. Fraysse, O. Deguine; volume co-editors, N. Cochard, R. Dauman, A. Uziel.
(Advances in oto-rhino-laryngology; vol. 48)
Includes bibliographical references and index. (alk. paper)
1. Cochlear implants – Congresses. 2. Deaf – Rehabilitation – Congresses.
3. Hearing impaired – Rehabilitation – Congresses.
I. Fraysse, Bernard G. II. Deguine, O. (Olivier) III. Series.
[DNLM: 1. Cochlear Implant – congresses. W1 AD701 v. 48 1993/WV 274 C6618 1992]
RF 16.A38 vol. 48 [RF305] 617.5'1 s--dc20 [617.8'82]
ISBN 3-8055-5767-1

Bibliographic Indices

This publication is listed in bibliographic services, including Current Contents® and Index Medicus.

Drug Dosage

The authors and the publisher have exerted every effort to ensure that drug selection and dosage set forth in this text are in accord with current recommendations and practice at the time of publication. However, in view of ongoing research, changes in government regulations, and the constant flow of information relating to drug therapy and drug reactions, the reader is urged to check the package insert for each drug for any change in indications and dosage and for added warnings and precautions. This is particularly important when the recommended agent is a new and/or infrequently employed drug.

Printed in Switzerland on acid-free paper by Thür AG Offsetdruck, Pratteln
ISBN 3–8055–5767–1

Contents

Surgical Techniques

Technical Failures

Coding Strategies

Electrophysiology

Results in Adults

Cochlear Implants in Children

Programming Techniques in Children

Educational Setting for Children

Results in Children

Different Systems

Preface

This book is the collection of some of the papers presented at the Symposium on Cochlear Implants: New Perspectives, held in Toulouse, June 2–3, 1992.

Over 400 participants from all over the world, representing many disciplines (speech therapists, neurophysiologists, physicians, ENT, neuroradiologists, engineers, psychologists, educators of the deaf, etc.), contributed to the success of this meeting.

Of the large number of papers submitted, due to lack of space, in most cases only the major contribution from each group was able to be published in this collection. The papers have been classified into areas of particular interest: basic science, patient selection, technical problems, surgical aspects, results in children and in adults.

In organizing this symposium and following it up by publication of this book, we hope to make a modest contribution to the progress made in this area since the first implant was produced by Djourno and Eyries in 1957, progress which has made cochlear implantation a reliable technique and an indispensable therapeutic alternative for profound or total deafness.

We would like to thank the authors for submitting to this publication papers presenting their most recent results. We would also like to express our thanks to the organisation committee, our secretaries, the Pierre Fabre Laboratories, and Cochlear AG, whose work, collaboration and support made the publication of this book possible.

Finally, we thank Karger Publishers for their help in preparing this book.

B. Fraysse

Inaugural Session

Fraysse B, Deguine O (eds): Cochlear Implants: New Perspectives.
Adv Otorhinolaryngol. Basel, Karger, 1993, vol 48, pp 1–3

Cochlear Implants: Past, Present and Future

William House

Newport Beach, Calif., USA

I have now been actively engaged in cochlear implant research for the past 34 years.

In Los Angeles the first wearable take home cochlear implant was produced by Jack Urban 20 years ago in 1972. Up to this time we had only stimulated our 2 volunteer patients for brief periods of time. I remember phoning the wife of our first patient, who was now using the implant 16 h a day, each day for several weeks to see if he could still hear. Many very knowledgeable researchers had predicted that the VIIIth nerve would soon give out if stimulated continuously. Each day that went by convinced Jack and I that we were on to something very exciting. Within a year, by implanting several more patients, we had a combined usage of 10 years of continuous stimulation. Amazingly, with over 3,000 patients worldwide using cochlear implants there have not been reports of VIIIth nerve failure. Today it seems very probable that a child implanted at age 2 will be able to use the implant for a lifetime of 70 or more years.

Today there is no longer any question that it works. There is no longer any question that these patients get timing, intensity and some frequency information. The early insistence that all these patients could possibly hear would be a Morse code like sound has now disappeared. The problem is that none of our neurophysiology colleagues have come forth with an explanation of how the implant works. This is a problem because it leaves us clinicians with no choice but trial and error to see if we can improve implant performance in our cochlear implant patients.

When Jack Urban and I started working with implants, I felt that discrete stimulation along the length of the basilar membrane would be necessary, so my first hard wired implants were 5 channel systems. Jack and I tried a number of frequency and filtering schemes with multi-band inputs. We also found that hooking all the electrodes together and using a 16-kHz amplitude carrier gave as good a result as the multiple channel inputs. This made no neurophysiological sense, but there it was.

At this point Jack and I were faced with a dilemma. Should we accept what the patient, Chuck Graser, was telling us, namely that the VIIIth nerve listens to the electric current it wants to hear, or should we say no we don't believe it because it makes no physiological sense.

We accepted what Chuck was telling us and thus the single-channel implant was born.

Subsequent temporal bone studies have shown that discrete limited electrical stimulation along the basilar membrane is not possible because the VIIIth nerve dendrites are missing. The only possible area of electrical stimulation is in the spiral ganglion. Indeed, it takes less current to reach electrical threshold with remote or common ground than with bipolar +1 stimulation. There is no neurophysiologic way of explaining, under these circumstances, how differences in intensity or frequency are attained. I have become a great believer in the concept that the VIIIth nerve and spiral ganglion listens to 'what it wants to hear'.

The Iowa 5-year randomized study using the 4-channel Utah Ineraid filtered 4 band signal, and the Cochlear Co. 22-channel feature extraction system showed no difference in the overall results. How can 2 such very different inputs give equal results? Do we listen to the patients or the neuropathologists?

At this time in the history of cochlear implants, I have become convinced that cochlear implants are 10% hardware and 90% software. By this I mean that the central nervous system has an amazing capacity to take whatever comes in over the VIIIth nerve and makes sense out of it. Some CNSs have more capacity to do this than others. This is the 90% software problem.

Hearing aid and implant research have shown us that reshaping of the external input can result in differences in patient performance. This is the 10% hardware problem.

And so we have learned that implants have the potential of lifetime rehabilitation of many thousands of deaf children and adults, that discrete electrical stimulation of small areas along the basilar membrane in the cochleas suitable for cochlear implants is not possible, and that the central nervous system is the most important factor in successful cochlear implant use. The question is 'Where do we go from here?'

I believe the next great need is for an implanted hardware system that will allow for the input of many different types of electronic analogs of sound. Although I have no personal experience with the system, I am told that the San Francisco system that is just being introduced will accomplish this need.

It is also possible to introduce all the variations of sound processing that are now possible in commercially available hearing aids through a single-channel implant. It is for this reason that I am reintroducing single-channel implant technology. My personal research in the next few years will be to explore the combination of single-channel implants and hearing aid technology.

Finally, in the future I see a great need for all of us as cochlear implant clinicians to insist that all future implant systems that are developed be simplified as much as possible.

I have no objection to developing and researching 4-, 8-, 22-, or even 50-channel implants, but once developed and tried on a number of patients, these complex systems must be researched to see if fewer channels can accomplish the same results.

Cochlear implants are here to stay. We must now continue to improve them. We must also simplify them as much as possible to make them available to all the deaf whose lives can be so greatly enhanced by their use.

Dr. William House, Hearing Associates, Newport Beach, CA 92658 (USA)

Basic Science

Fraysse B, Deguine O (eds): Cochlear Implants: New Perspectives.
Adv Otorhinolaryngol. Basel, Karger, 1993, vol 48, pp 4–8

Responses from Single Units in the Dorsal Cochlear Nucleus to Electrical Stimulation of the Cochlea

S.J. O'Leary, Y.C. Tong, G.M. Clark

Department of Otolaryngology, University of Melbourne, Parkville, Australia

An aim of the electrical stimulation strategy of a cochlear implant is to mimic the response of the auditory system to acoustic stimuli, so that hearing sensations generated by the implant can be recognisable and useful to the implantee. To help improve our understanding of how the brain responds to electrical stimulation of the auditory nerve we have examined the responses of dorsal cochlear nucleus (DCN) units to both acoustic and electrical stimulation of the cochlea in a hearing animal. This work extended our previous studies which have compared the responses to electrical and acoustic stimulation in the auditory nerve [1] and the ventral cochlear nucleus [2].

Our studies addressed two questions:

(1) What are the responses of DCN units to electrical stimulation of the auditory nerve?

(2) Was it possible to identify acoustic and electrical stimuli which generated similar responses from individual DCN units?

By answering questions 1 and 2, it may be possible to deduce the electrical stimulus parameters which should be employed in cochlear implant speech processing strategies to mimic acoustic-like responses from neurons of the dorsal cochlear nucleus. The generality of observations from the cochlear nucleus could then be tested at other nuclei within the central auditory pathways.

Methods

Single unit recordings were made from barbiturate-anaesthetised cats. The auditory nerve was activated by bipolar electrical stimulation of the cochlea using an electrode array similar to that used in the University of Melbourne-Cochlear Pty Ltd. Multiple Electrode Cochlear Implant. This stimulating electrode consisted of platinum bands mounted on a cylindrical carrier which fitted freely into the basal turn of the scala tympani and could be implanted without affecting the ABR thresholds to acoustic tone pips and clicks. The electrical stimulus was a 100-ms train of biphasic current pulses (100–200 μs/phase), delivered at 100–200 pulses/s. The stimulus current was 1.6–2.0 mA. The acoustic stimuli were 100-ms-duration acoustic tones and wideband noise at high stimulus intensity (93 dB SPL). The noise activated a broad cochlear region while the cochlear region activated by the characteristic frequency tone was less broad. The electrical stimulus, characteristic frequency tone and wideband noise stimuli were presented to each unit encountered. The poststimulus time histogram (PSTH) is the result of 50 presentations of the stimulus (presented every 400 ms).

Results

The envelope of the PSTH's in response to electrical stimulation exhibited 'primary-like' [3], 'onset' [3] or 'negative response' [4] and less frequently 'pauser' [3] or 'buildup' [4] patterns. Acoustic stimuli generate PSTH patterns with similar response envelopes [3, 4], and in this respect the range of DCN unit responses were similar in response to both acoustic and electrical stimuli. However, the action potentials in response to the electrical stimulus occurred in a narrow time window following each stimulus pulse and, therefore, were much less temporally dispersed than responses to acoustic stimuli. Note that responses of auditory nerve fibres [1] and ventral cochlear nucleus units [2] to electrical stimulation are much less temporally dispersed than responses to acoustic stimulation.

The second question was addressed in table 1. Each of the matrices summarises the incidence of PSTH patterns obtained from two stimuli (one acoustic and one electrical), and their interrelations. For example, the rows of the first matrix were the grouping of units into three major classifications, primary-like, negative response or onset (NR/O), pauser or buildup (P/B) according to their response to noise. The PSTH pattern grouping of the same unit to electrical stimulation is found in the columns. Units were counted if the discharge rate (during the stimulus) in response to *both* stimuli was within 50 spikes/s. Therefore, units were identified in which the responses to two types of stimulation were similar according to

Table 1. The number of units sharing the same PSTH pattern and a similar discharge rate in response to a 100-ms-duration electrical pulse train and a 100-ms-duration acoustic stimulus

Noise pattern	Electrical pattern			
	PL	NR/O	P/B	total
PL	6	2	1	9
NR/O	1	6	1	8
P/B	2	1	2	5
Total	9	9	5	23
CF tone pattern	**Electrical pattern**			
	PL	NR/O	P/B	total
PL	0	1	0	1
NR/O	3	5	3	11
P/B	3	0	0	3
Total	6	6	3	15
CF tone pattern	**Noise pattern**			
	PL	NR/O	P/B	total
PL	1	0	1	2
NR/O	0	5	0	5
P/B	3	0	0	3
Total	4	5	1	10

The stimulus intensity was high for both the acoustic and the electrical stimulus. The only units counted were those in which the discharge rate in response to both stimuli was within 50 spikes/s.
PL = A sustained response throughout the stimulus. For acoustic stimuli this corresponds with the chopper and primarylike PSTH patterns. For the electrical stimulus this meant that the P1 PSTH pattern was observed. NR/O = An onset or negative responser PSTH pattern to the stimulus; P/B = a pauser or buildup PSTH pattern to the stimulus.

both indices, PSTH pattern and discharge rate. From this analysis it was observed that responses to noise were similar to those from electrical stimulation in 14 of 32 units, but responses to a CF tone were similar to those from electrical stimulation less often (5 units of 32). It was concluded that, in hearing animals, the PSTH response to noise and electrical stimuli corresponded more frequently than the responses to electrical stimulation and a CF tone.

An essential control experiment was to demonstrate that the DCN responses recorded from hearing animals were due primarily to activation of the auditory nerve by the electrical stimulus, and not electrophonic mechanisms. This was tested by comparing DCN responses to electrical stimulation in hearing animals with those in animals deafened by neomycin irrigation of the scala tympani. The excitatory and inhibitory responses were very similar in hearing and deafened cats and, therefore, they were probably generated by the same mechanisms. Since electrophonic mechanisms were not active in the deafened animal the responses to electrical stimulation in both hearing and deaf animals were probably due to direct activation of the auditory nerve by the stimulus current. Thus there were reasonable grounds for using a hearing animal to contrast the responses of DCN units to acoustic and electrical stimulation of the auditory nerve, as performed in this study.

Conclusions

The PSTH and discharge rate responses to electrical stimulation and noise stimulation corresponded more frequently than the responses to electrical stimulation and CF tone stimulation. Therefore, some aspects of acoustic noise may be mimicked with a cochlear implant by presenting a high stimulus current, 100–200 pps pulse train. It is plausible that the correspondence of PSTH patterns and discharge rates in response to electrical stimulation and noise occurs because both stimuli activate a broad spatial extent of the cochlea.

References

1 Javel E, Tong YC, Shepherd RK, Clark GM: Responses of cat auditory nerve fibers to biphasic electrical current pulses. Ann Otol Rhinol Laryngol 1987;96:(suppl 128):26–30.

2 Shepherd RK, Xu SA, Williams JF, Maffi CL, Hatsushika S, Franz BK-HG, Tong YC, Clark GM, Millard RE, Wills RA, Kuzma JA, Patrick JF: Studies on paediatric auditory prosthesis implants. Fifth Quart Pro Report May-July 1988. NIH Contract NO1-NS-7-2342.
3 Pfeiffer RR: Classification of response patterns of spike discharges for units in the cochlear nucleus: Tone-burst stimulation. Exp Brain Res 1966;1:220–235.
4 Godfrey DA, Kiang NYS, Norris BE. Single unit activity in the dorsal cochlear nucleus of the cat. J Comp Neurol 1975;162:269–284.

Dr. Stephen J. O'Leary, Department of Otolaryngology, University of Melbourne, Parkville 3052 (Australia)

Fraysse B, Deguine O (eds): Cochlear Implants: New Perspectives.
Adv Otorhinolaryngol. Basel, Karger, 1993, vol 48, pp 9–16

A Study of Monopolar and Bipolar Stimulation Modes with a Modified Nucleus Mini-22 Cochlear Implant

Rolf-D. Battmer[a], *Detlev Gnadeberg*[a], *Ernst von Wallenberg*[b], *Ernst Lehnhardt*[a], *Dianne J. Allum*[b]

[a] Hals-, Nasen- und Ohrenklinik (Direktor: Prof. *T. Lenarz*), Medizinische Hochschule Hannover, BRD;
[b] Cochlear AG, Basel, Schweiz

Throughout the world nearly 7,000 subjects have already been supplied with a cochlear implant, nevertheless, research must continue in order to optimize existing systems and to develop more sophisticated ones. Useful hearing can only be achieved if the most important acoustic speech information is optimally converted to electrical stimulation parameters such as stimulation intensity, stimulation rate and stimulation place. For the design of smaller seized speech processors with more complex speech processing strategies, it is important to decrease the power consumption and to increase the stimulation rate.

Perception of electrical stimulation apparently does not take place through the dendrites but in the ganglion cells of the ganglion spirale [1]. This would suggest that a more radial spread of the electrical field – as in unipolar stimulation – might be more effective than a longitudinal one. Electrophysiological studies in cats [2] have demonstrated that the threshold for the firing of nerve fibres is about one third with unipolar stimulation than with a bipolar one. This means that the current for unipolar stimulation is much less than for bipolar stimulation. Shannon [3] showed that with a decrease in pulse width from 400 to 100 μs, loudness perception increases when the charge is kept constant. This suggests that to achieve similar loudness perception smaller pulse widths can be used. For pulse widths as low as 25 μs, this effect has not yet been studied. A reduction of pulse width, however, gives the possibility for increasing the stimulation rate.

To confirm these findings and to investigate further implications, a comparative study was designed. In the first part, the influence of unipolar and bipolar stimulation modes in terms of absolute identification of electrode rate and place pitch [4] and of speech perception performance was investigated. In a second study the effect of pulse width between 25 and 400 μs on threshold and maximum comfortable levels in both models was examined.

In both studies, a modified Mini-22 cochlear implant was needed which allowed the possibility to stimulate either in a bipolar or a unipolar mode. The Nucleus Mini-22 implant was modified into the Hannover Combi (fig. 1) implant in such a way that the intracochlear electrode array had only 20 active intracochlear electrodes. Electrode 1, an extracochlear remote ground electrode, is located next to the receiver-stimulator and is a partially exposed platinum wire wrapped around the standard electrode carrier. The Hannover Combi also has a single ball electrode on a free lead. In all subjects, it was placed near the round window; however, it was not activated during these experiments.

Programming of the speech processor was done in the normal fashion using an experimental version of the Nucleus software. For the study, 7 adult subjects were randomly selected and implanted with the Hannover Combi electrode array.

For the rate-pitch identification (fig. 2), the test electrodes were E5 and E17; each electrode received five different rates (126, 159, 200, 251 and 316 pps) presented at comfortable listening level. Before performing the psychophysical tests, equal loudness was estimated for all stimuli. The five stimuli were presented in random order. The confusion index [5] for 120 trials was calculated where a lower value represents few errors. The higher the index value, the more widely distributed and the further away from the target token are the answers. Subject 2 was unable to do the task with the apical electrode while subject 3 could identify pulse rates more reliably than all others. Altogether, no significant differences for rate-pitch identification could be observed in either mode.

For the place-pitch identification (fig. 3), five basal (E3, E5, E7, E9 and E11) and five apical (E11, E13, E15, E17 and E19) electrodes were chosen and used for both unipolar and bipolar conditions. The stimulation rate was fixed to 250 Hz; the pulse width was 200 μs. The test protocol for

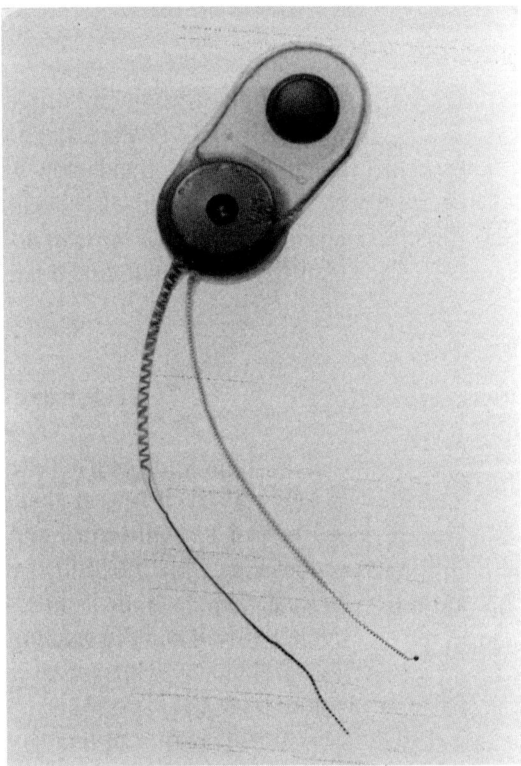

Fig. 1. The Hannover Combi Implant with 20 intracochlear banded and two remote electrodes. One remote electrode is located at the receiver/stimulator package and the other is a ball electrode, although implanted, was not used in this study.

this experiment was similar to the rate-pitch study. Only apical electrodes yielded a significant difference showing better results in bipolar mode ($p < 0.05$, Wilcoxon). There was an observable trend for lower index values suggesting that the bipolar-apical condition was the most easily identified.

For speech testing, several speech tests were administered after three months in unipolar mode, after another 3 months in bipolar mode and again after 3 months in unipolar mode. No significant differences were observed when comparing between all test interval scores with each other. All 6 subjects who joined the test showed a trend toward improvement over time when comparing only the unipolar mode.

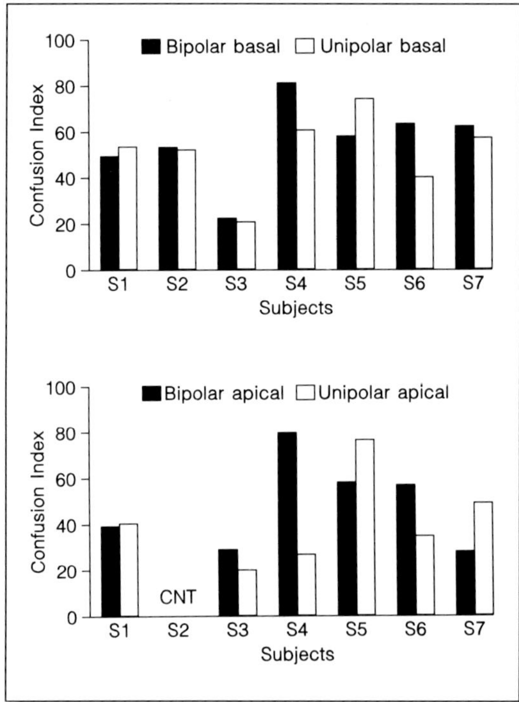

Fig. 2. Confusion index for rate pitch identification. Subject 2 could not do the task for the apical (E17) electrode, while subject 3 could identify rates much better than all other subjects.

To study the effect of pulse width on T and C levels, the current levels of the 7 subjects were evaluated for electrode 5 and 17 in unipolar and bipolar +3 mode; and for six different pulse width settings of 25, 50, 75, 100, 200 and 400 μs. In order to achieve equal loudness for all pulse width settings at C level, loudness balance was accomplished by comparing pairs of settings with different pulse widths and, finally, sweeping the full set of six.

For the analysis, only those 5 patients were taken who had data for all settings, including the difficult-to-reach C level for the 25-μs pulse width in bipolar mode. The current levels were converted into adjusted charge-per-phase (by the formula $Q = I \times PW$). The output current was obtained from the specific table for each implant, provided by the manufacturer. The

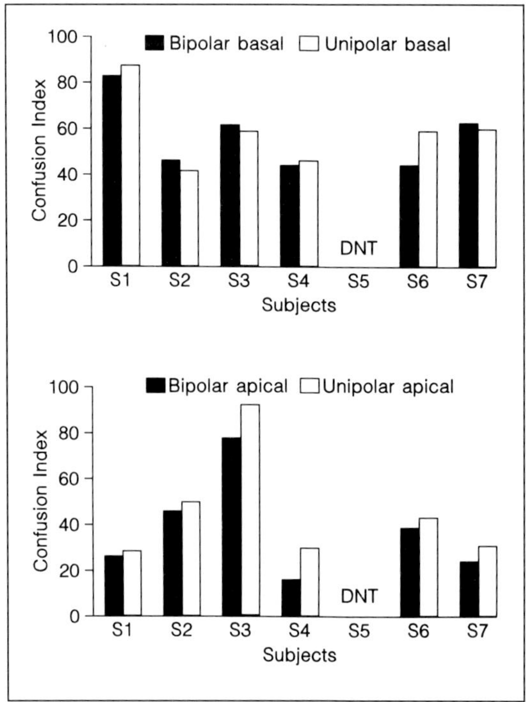

Fig. 3. Confusion index for place pitch identification. Subject 5 could not be tested due to facial nerve stimulation.

calculated charge values at T and C level were averaged separately for each electrode, for each pulse width and for both stimulation modes. All charge values were normalized to the value of the T level at 25 μs in unipolar mode and the mean dynamic range was calculated in dB.

It was found that the charge-per-phase (fig. 4) at threshold and maximum comfortable level in unipolar mode was approximately two and a half times less (1:2.4 = 7.6 dB) than in bipolar mode. This is in agreement with the findings of van den Honert and Stypulkowski [2], as mentioned earlier. The C level in unipolar mode is roughly equal to the T level in bipolar mode on both electrodes. The slope of the charge-per-phase versus pulse width was 2.5 dB per octave at T level and 3.2 dB per octave at C level and was similar for both modes. This confirms that lower pulse

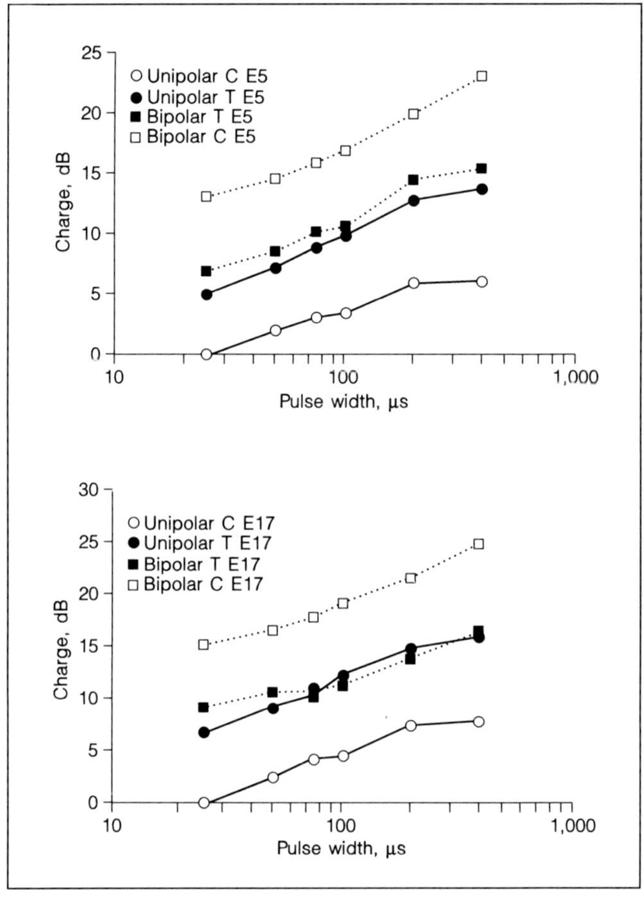

Fig. 4. Relative charge per phase for threshold (T) and maximum comfortable (C) levels versus pulse width. All values are normalized to the unipolar T level at 25 μs.

widths are more effective for producing auditory sensation [3]. In general, in unipolar mode the T and C levels appear to be more consistent across electrodes and the variance between patients was smaller. The average dynamic ranges (fig. 5), calculated in dB, however, are nearly the same in unipolar and in bipolar mode. As the pulse width increases from 75 to 400 μs, the dynamic range grows by approximately 2 dB. Below 75 μs the pattern seems to be more inconsistent.

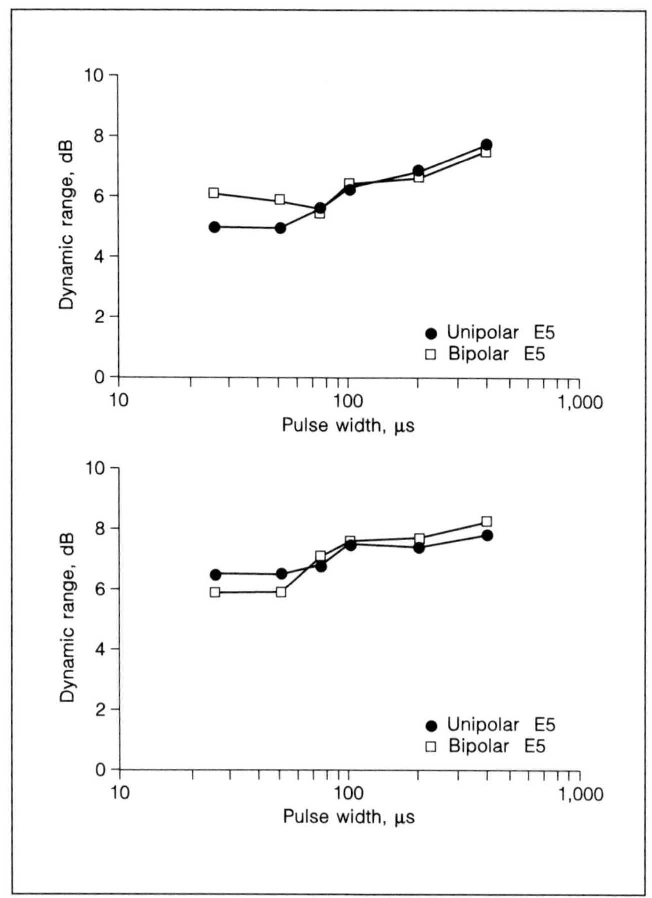

Fig. 5. Dynamic range versus pulse width. Above 75 μs the dynamic ranges are nearly equal in both modes.

Conclusions

In conclusion, it can be stated that all comparative tests between unipolar and bipolar stimulation modes show no significant differences, neither in rate and place pitch identification, in speech comprehension nor in dynamic range; only the place pitch identification test on the apical electrodes gave better results in bipolar mode. However, the smaller pulse width and the lower charge needed for equivalent auditory sensations in unipolar mode is more efficient. These findings should allow the development of new generations of speech processors with more sophisticated speech-processing strategies.

References

1 Linthicum FH, Galey FR: Histologic evaluation of temporal bones with cochlear implants. Ann Otol Rhinol Laryngol 1983;92:610–613.

2 van den Honert C, Stypulkowski PH: Single fiber mapping of spatial excitation patterns in the electrically stimulated auditory nerve. Hear Res 1987;29:195–206.

3 Shannon RV: Threshold and loudness functions for pulsatile stimulation of cochlear implants. Hear Res 1985;18:135–143.

4 Battmer RD, Gnadeberg D, von Wallenberg E, Lehnhardt E, Mecklenburg DJ: Comparative study of unipolar and bipolar stimulation modes with the Hannover Combi Mini-20+2 cochlear implant. J Acoust Soc A. Submitted.

5 Lai WK: Psychophysical studies investigating a place/rate coding strategy for a multiple-channel cochlear implant; PhD Diss, University of Melbourne 1990, pp 165–177.

Priv.-Doz. Dr. Rolf-D. Battmer, HNO-Klinik der Medizinischen Hochschule, Konstanty-Gutschow-Str. 8, D–30625 Hannover (FRG)

Patient Evaluation: New Perspectives

Fraysse B, Deguine O (eds): Cochlear Implants: New Perspectives.
Adv Otorhinolaryngol. Basel, Karger, 1993, vol 48, pp 17–22

Three-Dimensional Reconstruction of the Cochlea and Temporal Bone[1]

Markus C. Dahm[a,b], *H. Lee Seldon*[a], *Brian C. Pyman*[a], *Roland Laszig*[b], *Ernst Lehnhardt*[b], *Graeme M. Clark*[a]

[a] Department of Otolaryngology, University of Melbourne, The Royal Victorian Eye and Ear Hospital, East Melbourne, Victoria, Australia;
[b] HNO-Klinik und Poliklinik, Medizinische Hochschule Hannover, BRD

In recent years, cochlear implantation has become an established method for the auditory rehabilitation of profoundly deaf patients and is used in ever more and younger patients.

High-resolution computed tomography is performed routinely on all prospective cochlear implant patients and provides important information about cochlear or mastoid pathology that will enable the surgeon to select a side for operation and alert him to surgical obstacles he might encounter [1–4]. In analysing the CT films he must still try to form a three-dimensional image in his mind by looking through a large number of different pictures [5]. Consequently, to make it easier to understand, we applied our own image analysis system to produce three-dimensional reconstructions of temporal bones from CT scans [6]. We focused on the use of this method for the preoperative examination and surgical planning for cochlear implantation as well as for our research purposes. This system and the results are presented here.

[1] This work was supported by the NIH Contract NO1–NS–7–2342 Studies on Pediatric Auditory Prostheses Implants and a grant of the Deutsche Forschungsgemeinschaft DFG Da 232/1–2.

Methods

Input for the reconstructions can be any series of CT scans. The images are usually stored on X-ray films, but can also be saved on magnetic tapes or floppy discs. This information can easily be transferred to a personal computer. These video images are then digitized and stored on the personal computer. By transferring the image data onto our independent workstation, we overcome the problem of blocking valuable scanning time on the CT scanner computer. The program now allows the interpolation of a variable number of slices and either automatic, interactive or manual edge detection in the CT images. By selecting regions of interest on a particular scan, these features can be easily recognised in the following three-dimensional reconstruction. For instance, the ossicles, the round window and the facial recess can be highlighted by being plotted alone or in a different color than the surrounding structures. To enhance the three-dimensional appearance of the object shading can be added with a virtual light source from any angle and at any intensity. The most plastic three-dimensional appearance image, however, can be achieved by producing a video imitating rotation of the object. Within the display mode of the reconstruction program the user can rotate the object around all axes, zoom and move it, cut off a section at any level, or drill a hole to display otherwise hidden structures. In figure 1, the posterior part of a reconstructed temporal bone is cut off to show parts of the labyrinth and middle ear cleft with the ossicles.

By defining points of interest with the computer mouse, distances and angles can be calculated even after additional rotations, magnifications, drilling, etc. and can thereby provide important information for the surgeon planning the cochlear implant operation. This was used to determine the accuracy of our three-dimensional reconstruction system.

Results

The CT scan images of six cadaver temporal bones from children of different age groups were recorded, digitized and transferred onto our microcomputer. We selected several anatomical and surgical landmarks relevant for cochlear implant surgery in children, measured the distances between them using our reconstruction program and compared the calculated data with those yielded by direct calliper measurements after anatomical dissection of the same bones. The results show close correlation between the two sets of data, and we intend to use this method for the evaluation of the long-term effect that cochlear implantation may have on the growing skull. In 1991, we could harvest the temporal bone from an adult patient that died of unrelated cause several years after implantation. A CT scan was performed on this autopsy bone prior to histological processing. The resulting reconstructions are shown in figures 2 and 3.

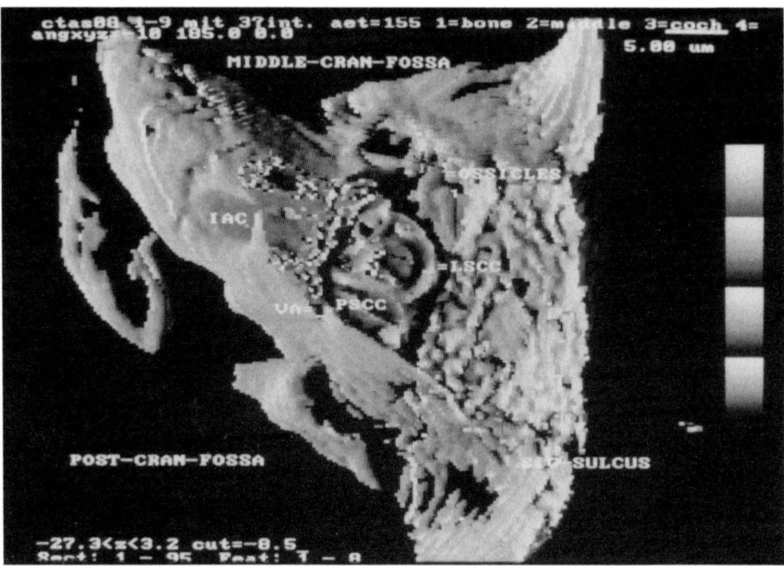

Fig. 1. Reconstructed image of a cadaver temporal bone with parts cut off to display otherwise hidden structures of the inner and middle ear.

In the reconstruction of the whole temporal bone you can easily see the mastoidectomy cavity and the electrode array in situ (fig. 2). By only displaying the electrode array, the ossicles and the inner ear spaces, the orientation of the implant inside the inner and middle ear becomes obvious (fig. 3).

In comparison to these postmortem studies, we could also reconstruct the temporal bone of a living implantee. In an 8-year-old child with a bilateral Mondini's malformation of the inner ear we performed a CT scan postoperatively and used this series for our reconstruction. Here also the receiver/stimulator is easily recognized. In the mastoid cavity the electrode array builds a loop to accommodate the expected growth of the skull and even the thin platinum wire used in Melbourne for the fixation of the electrode array at the fossa incudis is visible.

The presented system can be used without modification for the reconstruction of any set of serial section as MRI or histological sections. By connecting the video camera to a microscope we were able to examine a

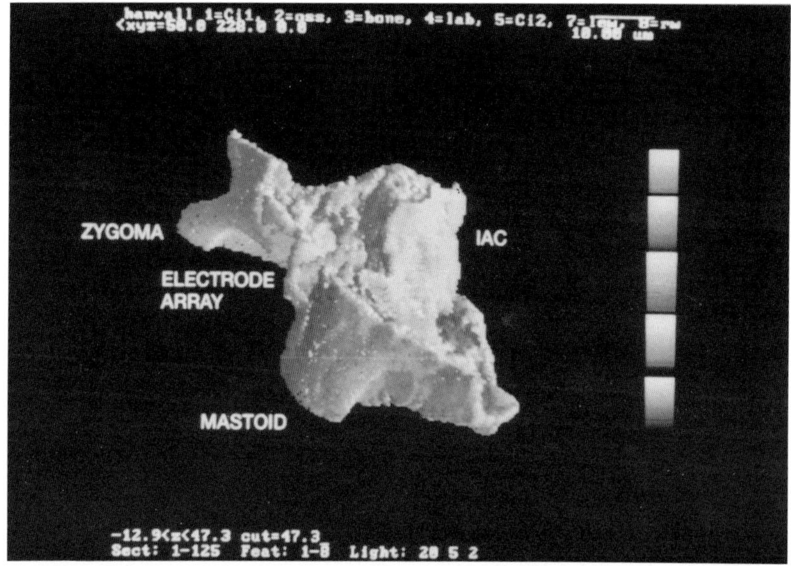

2

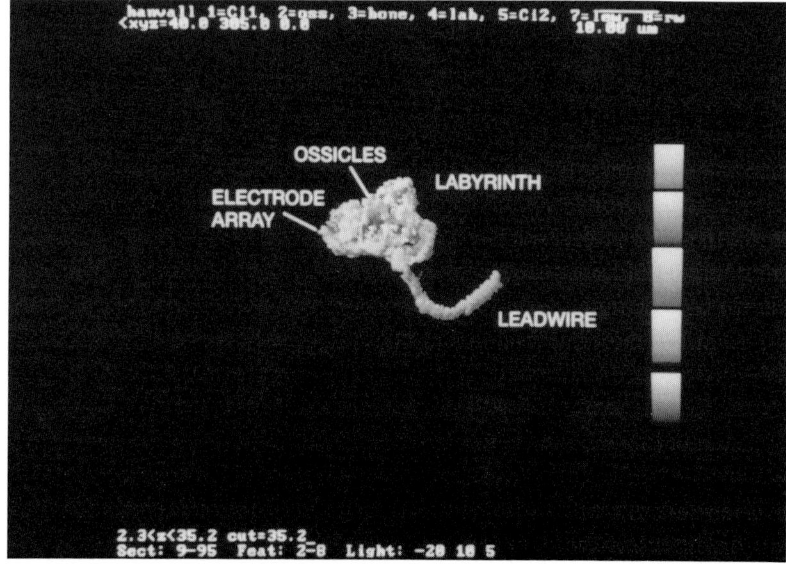

3

Fig. 2. Three-dimensional reconstruction of the cadaver temporal bone of a cochlear implant patient displaying the mastoidectomy cavity and the electrode in situ.

Fig. 3. The same object as in figure 2. Only the cochlear implant, the inner ear spaces and the ossicles are plotted, displaying the orientation of the electrode array in the inner and middle ear.

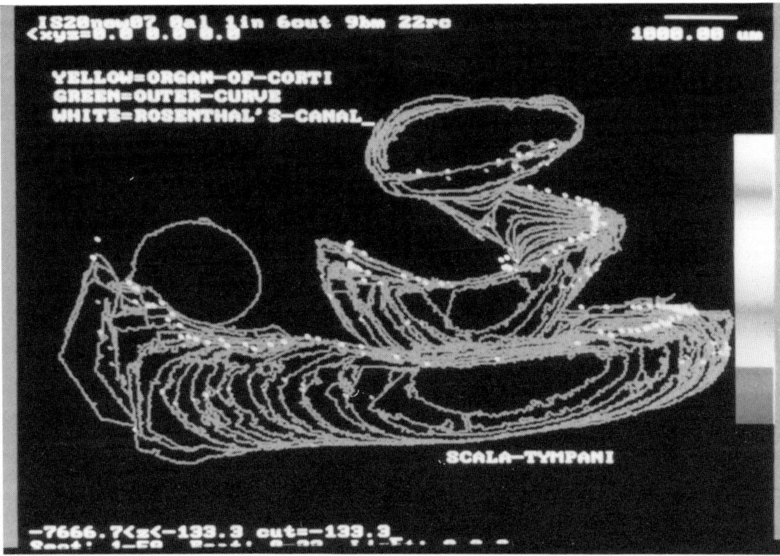

Fig. 4. Reconstruction of serial histology sections of a cochlea showing the spatial orientation of different structures.

series of histological sections of the cochlea. The resulting reconstruction is shown in figure 4.

The spatial relationship between the organ of Corti, the scala tympani and the spiral ganglion cells in Rosenthal's canal are visualized. Measurements along these structures can provide important information for future cochlear implant electrode design.

Discussion

By its nature the three-dimensional reconstruction can only detect features already present on the plain two-dimensional CT scan. But we believe it facilitates significantly the conceptualisation of the complicated anatomy of the ear and supplements plain CT scans. The presented program is an accurate and rapid method, providing helpful information for the implant surgeon and the researcher with interest in the anatomy of the temporal bone and cochlea.

References

1 Pyman BC, Brown AM, Dowell RC, Clark GM: Preoperative evaluation and selection of adults; in Clark GM, Tong YC, Patrick JF (eds): Cochlear Prostheses. Edinburgh, Churchill-Livingstone, 1990.

2 Phelps PD, Annis JAD, Robinson PJ: Imaging for cochlear implants. Br J Radiol 1990;63:512–516.

3 Harnsberger HR, Dart DJ, Parkin JL, Smoker WRK, Osborn AG: Cochlear implant candidates: Assessment with CT and MR imaging. Radiology 1987;164:53–57.

4 Mueller DP, Dolan KD, Gantz BJ: Temporal bone computed tomography in the preoperative evaluation for cochlear implantation. Ann Otol Rhinol Laryngol 1989; 98:346–349.

5 LaRouere MJ, Niparko JK, Gebarski SS, Kemink JL: Three-dimensional x-ray computed tomography of the temporal bone as an aid to surgical planning. Otolaryngol Head Neck Surg 1990;103:740–747.

6 Seldon HL: 3-D reconstruction of temporal bone from CT scans on a personal computer. Arch Otolaryngol Head Neck Surg 1991;117:1158–1161.

Dr. Markus C. Dahm, Department of Otolaryngology, University of Melbourne,
The Royal Victorian Eye and Ear Hospital, 32 Gisborne Street,
East Melbourne, Vic. 3002 (Australia)

Fraysse B, Deguine O (eds): Cochlear Implants: New Perspectives.
Adv Otorhinolaryngol. Basel, Karger, 1993, vol 48, pp 23–28

Place of 3DFT-MR Imaging Study on Cochlear Implant Candidates

K. Marsot-Dupuch[a], *Ch. Chouard*[b], *B. Falisse*[c], *B. Meyer*[b], *J.M. Tubiana*[a]

Departments of [a]Radiology (Prof. *J.M. Tubiana*) and
[b]Head and Neck (Prof. *Ch. Chouard*), St. Antoine's Hospital, Paris;
[c]Department of Biomedicine, Siemens France, Saint Denis, France

The ability to predetermine the auditory benefit of a cochlear implant device in patients with severe hearing loss is limited. Choice between a multicanal or a monocanal device and of its intra- or extracochlear location is to a great deal due to their different prices and results. It depends upon a number of factors such as permeability of the basal turn of the cochlea. Our purpose was to establish the capacity of a 3DFT-MR sequence compared to CT and convertional MRI to evaluate labyrinthine liquid status, internal auditory canal, and size of acoustic nerve, and to detect ear malformation. All these factors predict the surgical success of cochlear implantation.

Material and Methods

Material

After undergoing routine clinical and paraclinical evaluation, 24 pre-implant candidates underwent imaging studies from March 1991 to May 1992. Ages ranged from 7 to 60 years. Four patients were excluded from the study due to the insufficient image quality (2 cases), a previous ear device (1 case) and the early age of a young patient needing premedication for MRI. Eight of 20 patients underwent surgery. The surgical data were correlated to the imaging study.

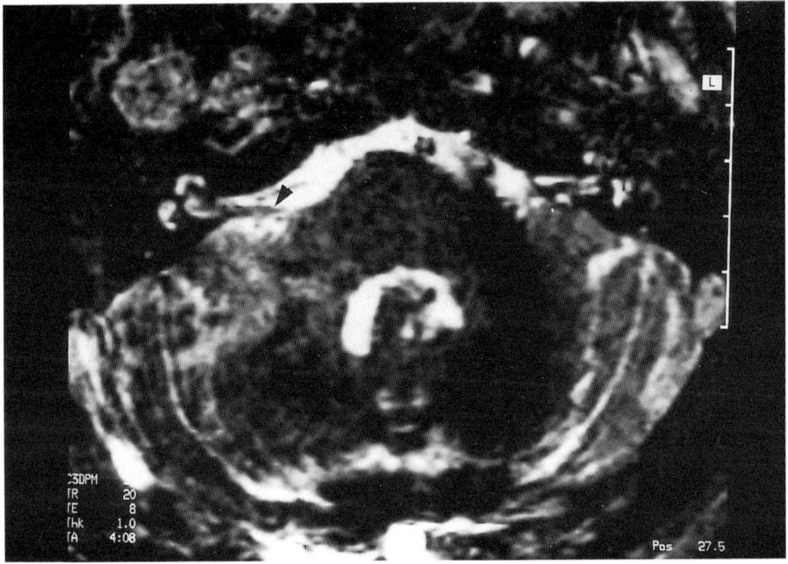

Fig. 1. MRI, CISS sequence, lower part of the IAC. High signal intensity of the pontocerebellar angle CSF. Delineation of each nerve (arrowhead): note the cochlear nerve anteriorly and the inferior vestibular nerve posteriorly. High signal intensity of labyrinthine fluid showing cochlea, vestibule and semicircular canals.

Methods

To assess the status of middle ear, mastoid and cochlear patency, the patients were screened by both CT and MRI examinations. We classically used thin (1 mm) axial contiguous sections of high resolution CT (Somaton plus) without iodine injection, done in the orbito-meatal plane. Coronal contiguous sections were obtained in 21 tolerant patients. All MR examinations were performed on a 1 T Siemens unit with a head coil, allowing simultaneous bilateral and comparative examinations. 3-mm contiguous axial sections pre- and postgadolinium T1 weighted images (WI) (TR: 500 ms; TE: 20 ms). T2 WI were acquired using *both* a standard spin-echo sequence (TR 2,200 ms, TE 120 ms) (8 min long, 5 mm thickness) and a T2 WI 3-DFT sequence (5 min long, 1 mm thickness). This last short gradient echo sequence, called CISS (constructive interference study state) is potentially useful for delineating CSF and labyrinthine liquid due to its inherent high T2 contrast, comparable to long TR/long TE convertional spin echo sequence. As it is 3D acquisition, the resolution is high. Its parameters are: TR 50 ms, TE 20 ms, flip angle 50°, matrix 256 × 256, FOV 180 mm, ACQ 1, SLAB 32, acquisition time 2 × 2 mm 46 s, plane resolution 0.69 × 0.69. The application of symmetrical flow compensated to correct the CSF motion to which this sequence is very sensitive. After processing of these thin contiguous sections by a 'maximun intensity projection' (MIP), 3D images of the inner ear structures are able to be made.

Fig. 2. 3D reconstruction. Good delineation of the basal turn of the cochlea (arrow), vestibule and semicircular canals (arrowhead).

Results

Thanks to the high signal intensity of the endo- and perilabyrinthine fluid and the extreme thin section thickness. CISS images allow an excellent delineation of the labyrinthine structure. Each nerve of the internal auditory canal is exquisitely delineated in the CSF (fig. 1). In all patients, the anatomy of the labyrinthine structures was depicted. This sequence enabled us, thanks to the 3D reconstruction of the membranous labyrinth, to turn the labyrinth 360°, and allowed us to look for the diameter and the permeability of the basal turn of the cochlea (fig. 2) thereby detecting focal areas of fibrous deposits. In 5 of 7 patients who underwent surgery, the diagnosis and site of fibrous obliteration of the endo- and perilymphatics was made possible by CISS images, therefore predicting the success of the cochlear implant in advance (fig. 3). This obliteration of the labyrinthine fluid was due to meningitis (3 cases, 1 case bilateral), cochlear otosclerosis (1 case), and posttrauma (1 case). In all patients except one with otospongiosis, T1 MR was considered normal. Spin-echo T2 WI was only

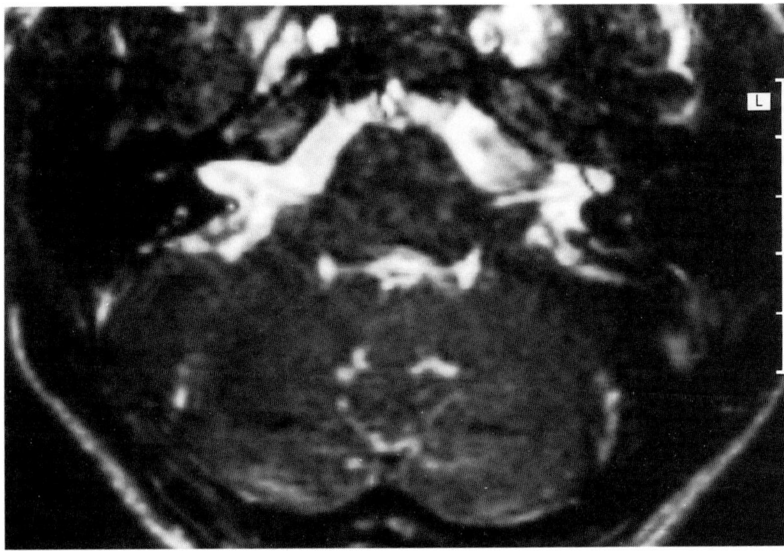

Fig. 3. MRI, CISS sequence. Loss of the normal high signal intensity of both labyrinths due to ossification on the left side and fibrous deposits on the right side. Large internal auditory canal with a vascular loop in the left side.

positive in 3 cases and was insufficient to clearly demonstrate extension of the obliteration. CT failed to detect cochlear obliteration in 3 cases (1 cochlear otosclerosis, 1 meningitis, 1 trauma). Moreover, the CISS sequence delineates the internal auditory canal (IAC) showing us a vascular loop in the IAC in 10% of the patients as the high signal intensity of the CSF contrasts with the low signal intensity of the nerves and the surrounding bone. Stenosis of the IAC was depicted in 1 patient by both CT and MRI.

The CISS sequence failed to depict middle ear aeration and mastoid pneumatisation and a middle ear cholesteatoma was overlooked. A case of cochlear otospongiosis, well-depicted by CT and suspected by the T1 WI sequence, was misdiagnosed by the CISS sequence as no modification of the labyrinthine fluid was present. Artefacts due to movements and to magnetic susceptibility explain 7% of the insufficient quality images.

Discussion

The presurgical status of the implant candidates [1] rules out several kinds of answers: What is the status of the mastoid and middle ear aeration? What is the status of the endo- and perilabyrinthine fluid? What is the size of the internal auditory canal and how are the nerves inside? CT [2] remains the best method for presurgical bone evaluation delineating the mastoid pneumatisation and the middle ear aeration status, and detecting occult infection of the middle ear consisting of a contraindication to surgery. If it depicts cochlear ossification and the modification of the surrounding bone well, it fails to depict early labyrinthine changes due to fibrous deposits. Meanwhile, 3DFT-MR is the procedure of choice for evaluating the permeability of the labyrinthine fluid, showing in advance fibrous obliteration of the labyrinth, its amount and its location. Thanks to the 1-mm thick slices obtained by 3D imaging, size of the basal turn of the cochlea, of the internal acoustic canal and of the cochlear nerve can be appreciated. T2 WI are the only way of detecting brain atrophy or any occult damage along the acoustic pathway, thereby predicting failure of the implant device in advance.

Conclusion

Our preliminary report demonstrates the value of 3DFT-MR to appreciate the labyrinthine fluid thanks to its high signal intensity excluding fibrotic obliteration. It adds important information for evaluation of membranous labyrinthic pathologies in implant candidates. Early detection of membranous obliteration and evaluation of its degree and location help when planning implant surgery, determining the size to operate, choice of the type of implant (monocanal versus multicanal) [3], and the intra- or extracochlear location of the device. CT remains unrivaled for depicting the degree and the quality of middle ear aeration and for follow-up of implant surgery as MRI is definitely contraindicated. CT and 3DFT-MR now appear both necessary in the presurgical study of implant candidates, especially if the price of multicanal implants is considered. Postgadolinium T1 WI are not useful, except in some rare cases where precise detection of labyrinthine membrane abnormalities should be a key point to decide the time of surgery.

References

1 Fugain C, Chabolle F, Meyer B, Chouard C: Résultats cliniques de l'implant cochléaire multi-électrode dans la réhabilitation de 24 cas de surdité totale acquise. Ann Otol Laryngol 1988:105:253–259.

2 Wiet R, Pyle M, O'Connor C, Russel C, Schramm DR: Computed tomography: How accurate a predictor for cochlear implantation. Laryngoscope 1990;100:687–690.

3 Franz B, Kusma J, Lehnhard J, Clark G, Patrik J, Laszi JR: Implantation of the Melbourne cochlear multiple electrode extracochlear prothesis. Ann Otol Rhinol Laryngol 1989;98:591–596.

Dr. K. Marsot-Dupuch, Department of Radiology, St-Antoine's Hospital, 184, rue du Faubourg-St-Antoine, F–75012 Paris (France)

Fraysse B, Deguine O (eds): Cochlear Implants: New Perspectives.
Adv Otorhinolaryngol. Basel, Karger, 1993, vol 48, pp 29–34

Auditory Cortex Activities in Severely Hearing-Impaired and Cochlear Implant Patients

Positron Emission Tomographic Study

Juichi Ito

Department of Otolaryngology, Otsu Red Cross Hospital, Otsu, Siga, Japan

Over the past 5 years, we have performed Australian multi-channel cochlear implantation [1] in 24 patients.

Even though the implant device provides insufficient information, the speech comprehension of cochlear implant patients is fairly good [2]. The higher brain system has been presumed to play an important role in the discrimination of speech. The purpose of the study presented here was to investigate the function of the auditory cortex in severely hearing-impaired and deaf patients. In this study, we used positron emission computed tomography (PET), which allows monitoring of brain activity, because it provides quantitative measurements of oxygen and glucose metabolism [3].

In some cochlear implant patients, we performed PET both before and after cochlear implant operation; these data can be analyzed to assess functional changes of the auditory cortex.

Materials and Methods

We used a whole-body, multi-slice PET, Positologica III, in this study. The positron-releasing chemical 18F-fluoro-deoxyglucose (FDG) was used to measure local changes in cerebral glucose metabolism [4].

Table 1 shows the clinical characteristics of the patients in whom PET was performed (total = 12).

Table 1. Clinical characteristics of the patients in whom PET was performed

Patient No.	Age	Sex	Cause of deafness	Period of deafness, years
1	26	F	otosclerosis	5
2	41	M	sudden deafness	3
3	42	M	head injury	1
4	51	M	meningitis	1
5	39	M	labyrinthitis	1
6	53	M	meningitis	2
7	52	F	unknown	5
8	54	F	Menière's disease	10
9	59	M	Menière's disease	10
10	61	M	streptomycin	25
11	58	F	sudden deafness	25
12	38	M	streptomycin	37

The patients were divided into two groups on the basis of whether they were severely hearing-impaired (patients 1 and 2) or totally deaf (patients 3–12). In addition, the totally deaf patients were divided into those who had been deaf for a relatively short period of time (patients 3–7) or for a long period of time (patients 8–12).

Patients 1, 3, 4, 5, 8, 9, 11 and 12 underwent cochlear implant surgery. Three of these patients (patients 4, 9 and 12) underwent PET both before and after surgery. Postoperative PET was performed during auditory stimulation.

Results

Figure 1 shows the PET images of patient 1. The patient is an example in the first group with some residual hearing. The patient was a 26-year-old female who first noticed hearing disturbance at the age of 12. The disturbance progressively worsened and she became markedly deaf 4 or 5 years before cochlear implantation. The audiogram indicated that there was some residual low-frequency hearing. The PET image appears to be almost normal, even though the audiogram before operation did not reveal good response to sound. The PET image of another patient (patient 2) with residual hearing was also almost normal.

Figure 2 shows the PET images for patient 3. The patient is an example for patients in the second group, that is, the patients who had been deaf

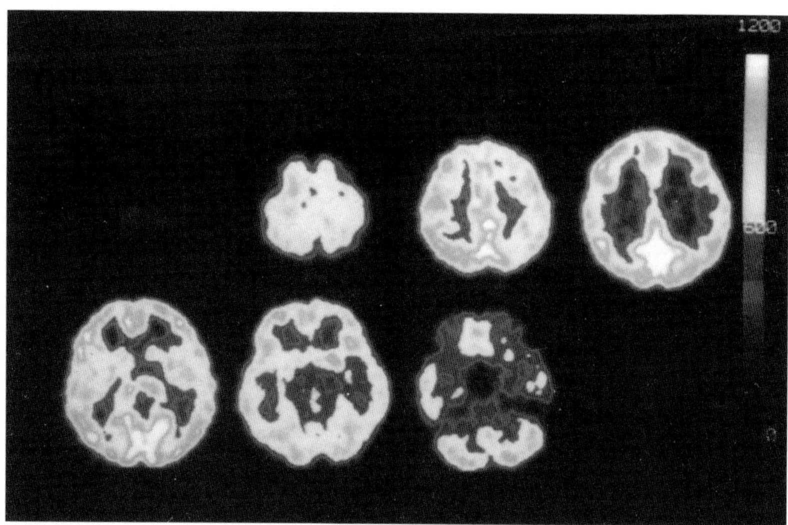

Fig. 1. PET image of patient 1.

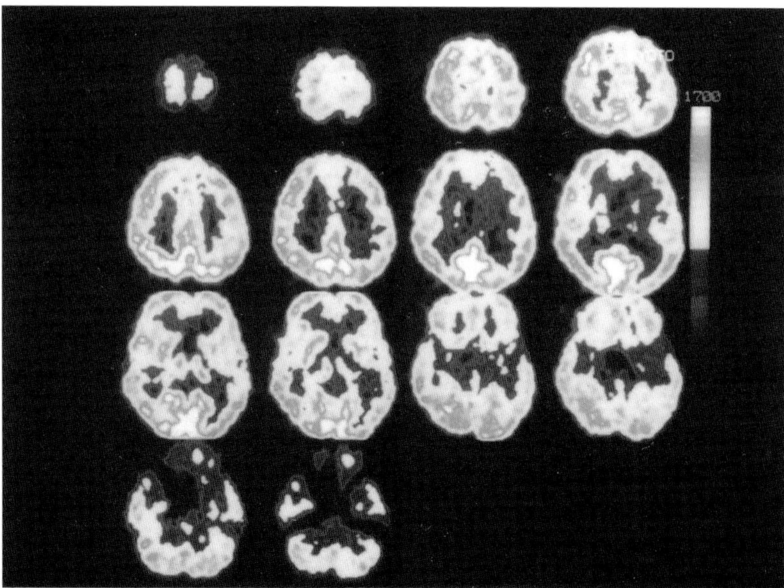

Fig. 2. PET image of patient 3.

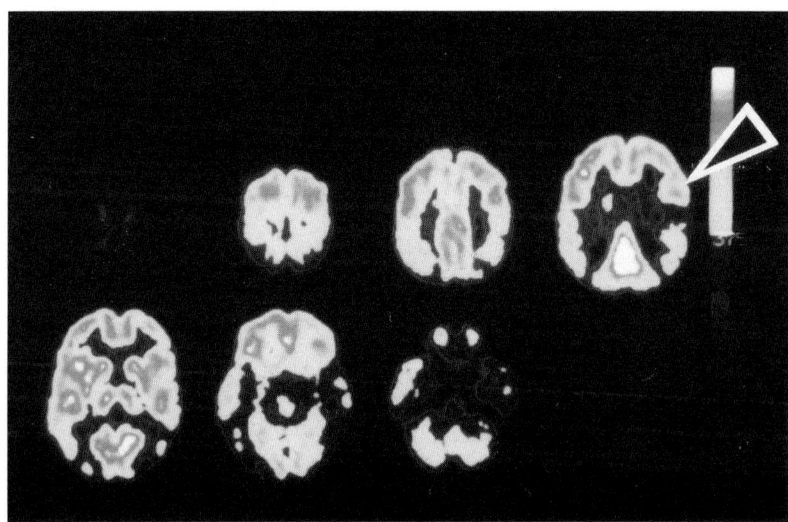

Fig. 3. PET image of patient 12 (before cochlear implantation). PET image demonstrating cerebral glucose metabolism in the control state. Arrows show the low activity areas.

for a relatively short period of time. Pure tone audiogram demonstrated that he was totally deaf. The patient was a 42-year-old male who fell from a height of 5 m and was diagnosed as having temporal bone facture on the basis of high-resolution CT. He became totally deaf 1 year before cochlear implantation. The PET images of this patient shows that there is slight decrease of the metabolic rate in bilateral primary auditory cortices, but as such changes can often be observed in persons with normal hearing, this PET image was considered to be almost normal or showed slight decrease.

Patient 12 is an example in the last group and had been deaf for a long period of time. The patient was a 38-year-old male who, because of lung tuberculosis, was given streptomycin at the age of 1 year and became almost deaf several months later. This patient was a so-called prelingual deaf patient. He underwent cochlear implantation, and we compared PET images before and after operation.

Figure 3 shows the preoperative PET images for this patient. The PET images show that, preoperatively, there was a markedly low metabolic rate in the primary auditory cortex and in some of the associate cortices. Figure 4 shows the postoperative PET images, which were obtained during

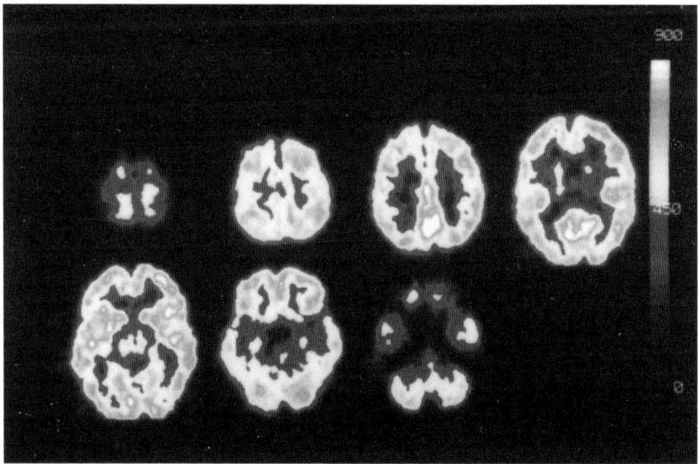

Fig. 4. PET image of patient 12 (after cochlear implantation). The low activity areas on the left, which were visible before the operation, have almost disappeared.

auditory stimulation. The patient had been instructed to listen carefully to the sound stimulation.

The metabolic rate in the primary and secondary cortices returned to near normal levels.

Discussion

The results of the present study show that PET findings for patients with residual hearing are almost normal and it can be concluded that, in patients with residual hearing, the activity of the auditory cortex measured by PET is almost normal.

As for the deaf patients, the metabolic rate in the auditory cortex in patients who have been deaf for a short period of time is almost normal or slightly decreased.

On the other hand, the patients who have been deaf for a long time show decreased activity in the auditory cortex. We can conclude that if the period of deafness is long, that is, if it exceeds 10 years, not only the primary auditory cortex but also the secondary associate cortex will show low metabolic rate.

We also compared the PET findings with speech comprehension ability. While the number of patients in the present study was too small for us to draw any firm conclusions, our results do suggest that patients with normal PET images show fairly good speech comprehension following cochlear implant operation, while patients with very low metabolic rate in the auditory cortex detected using PET often show moderate or poor speech comprehension. This result suggests that it may be possible to predict speech comprehension ability from PET prior to cochlear implant surgery.

References

1 Clark GM, Tong YC, Bailey QR, Black RC, Martin LF, Millar JB, et al: A multiple-electrode cochlear implant. J Otolaryngol Soc Aust 1978;4:208–212.
2 Ito J, Tsuiji J, Sakakibara J, Takeuchi M, Honjo I: Studies on speech perception by multiple cochlear implant. Studia Phonol 1989;22:50–55.
3 Ell PJ, Holman BL (eds): Computed Emission Tomography. New York, Oxford University Press, 1982, pp 1–239.
4 Senda M, Tamaki N, Yonekawa Y, Tanada S, Murata K, Hayashi N, et al: Performance characteristics of positiologica. III. A wholebody positron emission tomograph. J Comput Assist Tomogr 1985;9:940–946.

Juichi Ito, MD, Department of Otolaryngology, Otsu Red Cross Hospital,
Otsu, Siga 520 (Japan)

Fraysse B, Deguine O (eds): Cochlear Implants: New Perspectives.
Adv Otorhinolaryngol. Basel, Karger, 1993, vol 48, pp 35–43

The Contribution of Brain Mapping in the Wearer of a Cochlear Implant

Preliminary Report

M. Gersdorff, J.M. Guerit, N. Deggouj, M. de Tourtchaninoff

University of Louvain, Cliniques Universitaires St Luc, Brussels, Belgium

The purpose of this paper is to present you with the first results, and with our interpretation, of brain mapping in the wearer of a Nucleus type cochlear implant.

It will be remembered that 'brain mapping' and 'electrocartography' are the terms used for the recording of evoked cortical potentials by means of 20 electrodes placed on the scalp according to the International 10–20 system.

Examination takes place by means of Nicolet BEAM I: binaural stimulation by 25 ms tone bursts at 1,000 Hz, with a rise and decay of 10 ms, an analysis time of 1,024 ms, 200 responses averaged 3 times with a pseudo-random rate of 0.7 Hz.

The late auditory evoked potentials are constituted by three peaks [4], designated P I, N I and P II of which the peaks N I at about 100 ms (= N 100) and P II at about 180–200 ms (= P 200), are habitually studied.

These evoked auditory potentials may be considered as *exogenous,* i.e. essentially influenced by the characteristics of external stimulation applied to the individual.

In brain mapping, the distribution of these evoked cortical potentials in the normal subject are median and symmetrical (fig. 1). In the case of binaural stimulation, the temporal generators do indeed simultaneously charge themselves symmetrically; the vectorial resulting from these two symmetric temporal dipoles will be median [1–3]. However, in the case of unilateral stimulation, or in that of unilateral lesion of the auditory cortex, the bilateral temporal cortex being no longer stimulated in an identical and

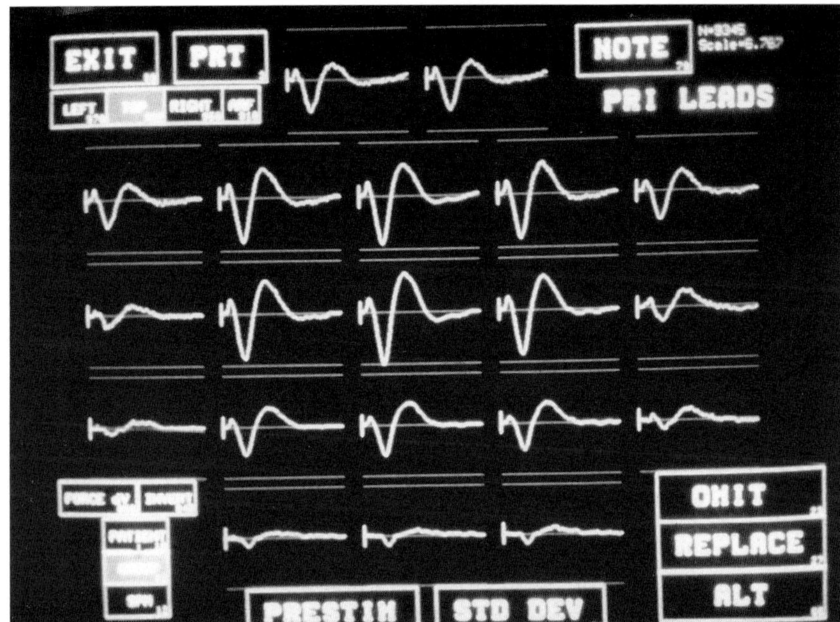

a

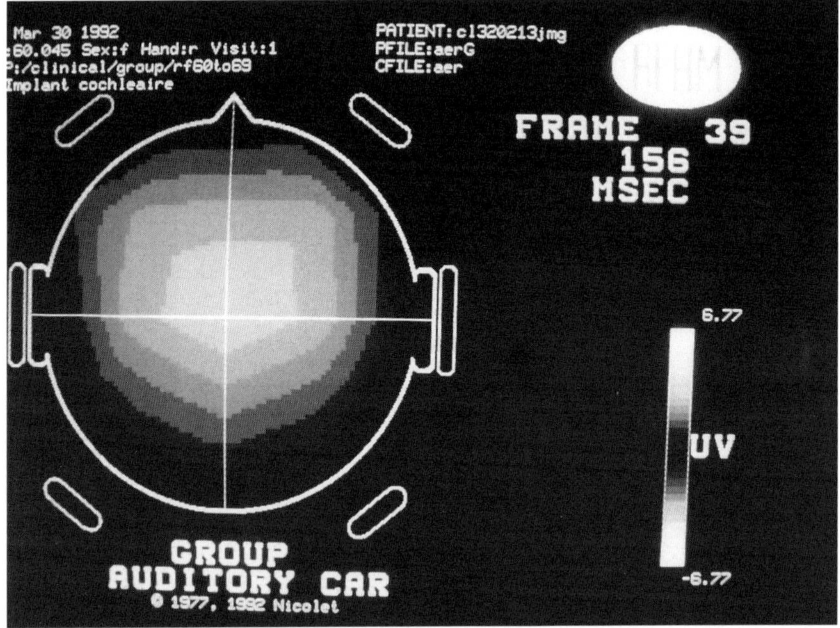

b

Fig. 1. Brain mapping. Normal late auditory evoked potentials obtained by binaural stimulation.

symmetrical manner, the resulting vector will be lateralized towards the health side.

It should be noted that, because of the main crossing-over of the auditory pathways in the case of unilateral stimulation, the response by the scalp is controlateral.

The evoked potentials as a whole no longer depending simply on physical characteristics but on the reaction of the subject confronting the stimulation, are regrouped under the term of endogenous or cognitive evoked potentials, these including the P 300 wave [4].

Supposing that one presents a series of tone bursts constituted on the one hand by 1,000 Hz stimuli in 90% of the cases and, on the other hand, of 1,500 Hz stimuli in 10% of the cases, and that the subject is told to press a button or to raise his hand each time there is stimulation to 1,500 Hz, i.e. a rare stimulation, we see, on the one hand, N I and P II exogenous evoked potentials but, during the rare stimulation, a positive wave of great amplitude that can reach 20 μV and a latency time in the order of 300 ms, the P 300.

The functional significance of the P 300 is not well understood; one might say it is the expression of a certain recognition, auditory in the present instance, an indicator of perception by sensorial stimuli.

Substraction of the curves obtained confirms the existence of the P III–N III complex, thus of the P300, endogenous cognitive evoked potentials.

To be noted also is the existence of an N II wave, N 200 preceding the wave P300 and named 'mismatch negativity'.

Five adult patients having worn a Nucleus cochlear implant for more than 1 year have been examined by brain mapping.

(1) Electric stimulation via the cochlear implant (pulse rate: 250 Hz; pulse duration: 100 ms; interstimulus: 1,000 ms) [5] has proved to be a failure. We are essentially observing electric artefacts. The results are not reproducible. A technique for dephasing electric stimulations is being studied and could perhaps provide satisfactory results.

(2) In contrast, by *acoustic stimulation* using tone bursts, at 1,000 Hz in this first preliminary study, for the speech processor of the cochlear implant, we obtain evoked auditory potentials by brain mapping, with results that vary from one individual to another.

The results do not seem to have any relation with the performance of the patients. For none of the patients tested can the curves obtained be considered normal, not even for our 'star' patients. Figure 2a presents the

a

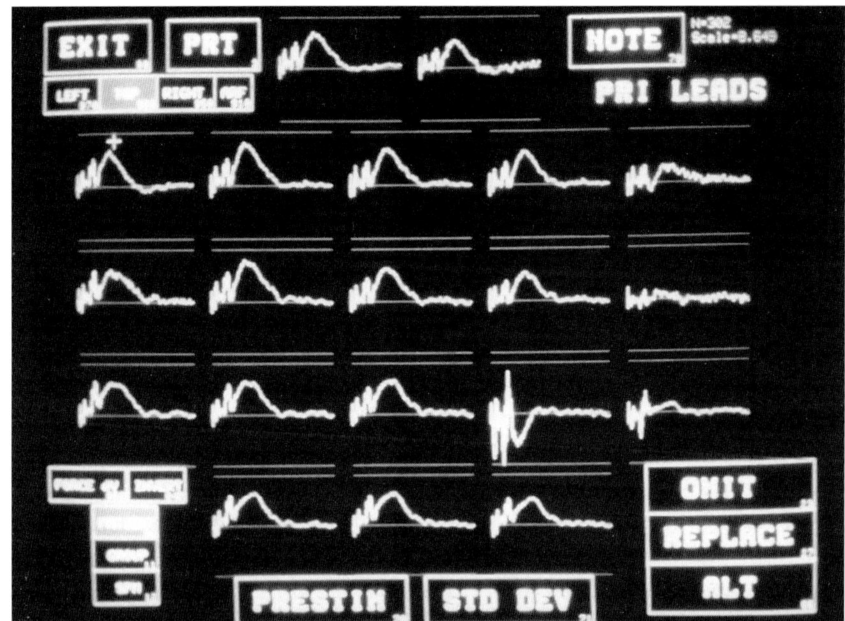

b

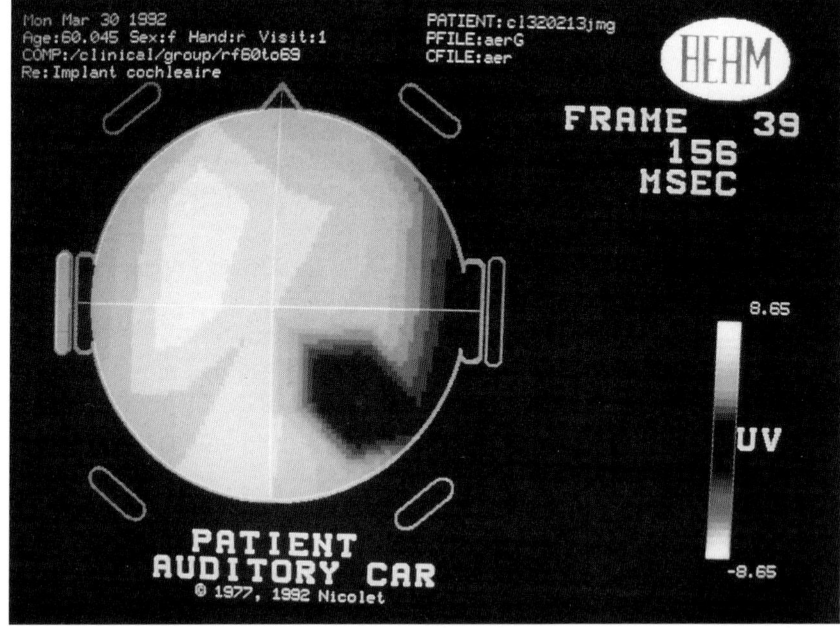

Fig. 2. Brain mapping. Late auditory evoked potentials. Right cochlear implant. Acoustic stimulation: 1,000 Hz tone bursts (see text).

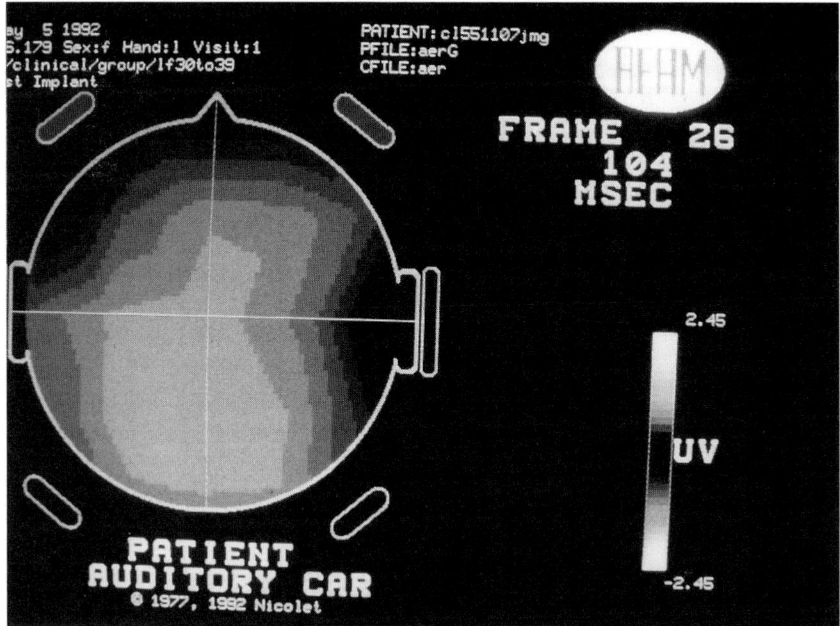

a

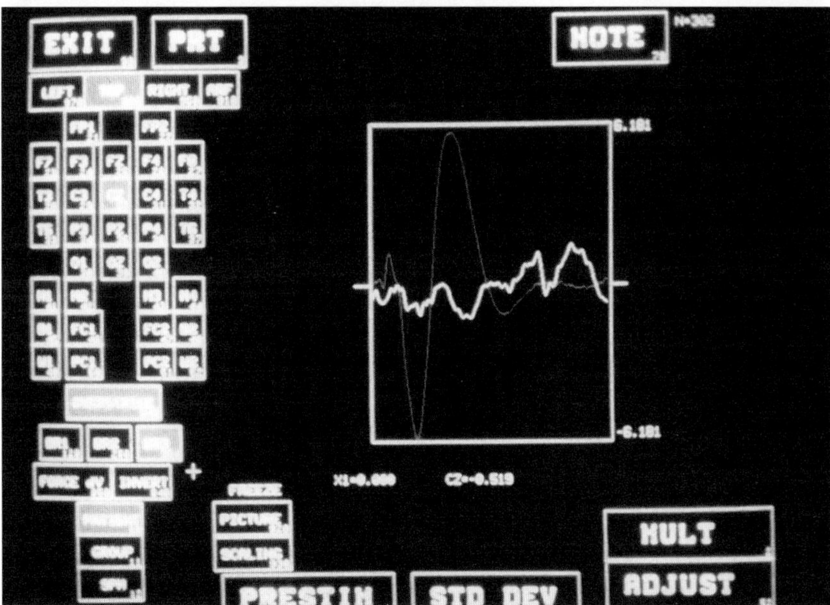

b

Fig. 3. Brain mapping. Late auditory evoked potentials. Cochlear implant. Acoustic stimulation: 1,000 Hz tone bursts (see text).

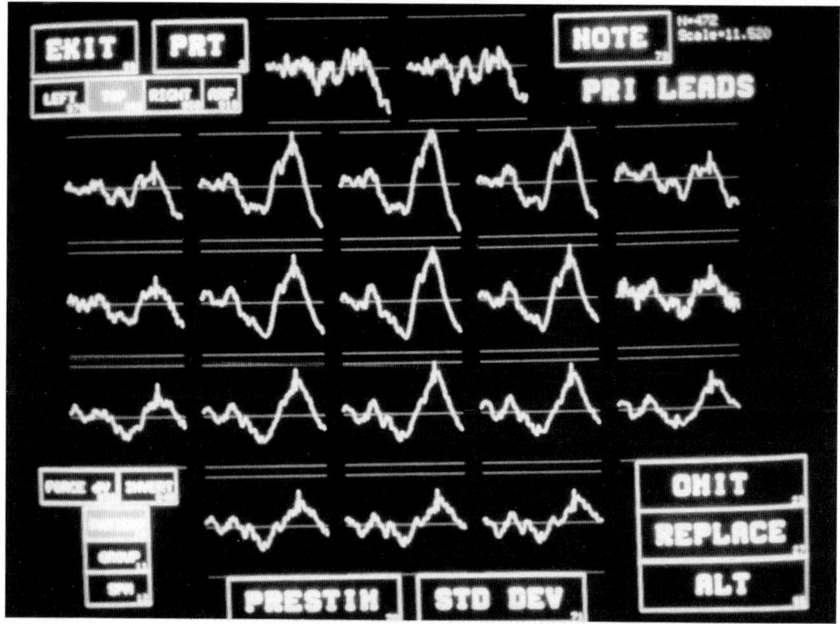

Fig. 4. Brain mapping. Same patient as in figure 3. Cognitive evoked potentials (1,000–1,500 Hz).

results of 1 patient. You will note to the right a large stimulation artefact at the side where the cochlear implant is situated.

Later, we can observe a positive response at 150 ms with a maximum of responses in the frontal and controlateral temporal derivations.

In the same patient, by cartography (fig. 2b) you observe the electric artefact as darkest, and a maximum of front-central, contralateral activities as lightest. Note that the curves are less well-synchronized than in the normal subject (fig. 1).

The topography and the morphology of the response are abnormal.

Figure 3a presents another patient, a star patient. His tracings are anarchic and continually changing. This is an example at 104 ms. The gradient is very blurred, the amplitude in the order of 2 μV. Nothing can be concluded from this type of curve, except that there is cortical activation, but it is anarchic and does not correspond to any known pattern.

In figure 3b you will see the cortical auditory activities of this patient compared to the response from a normal subject.

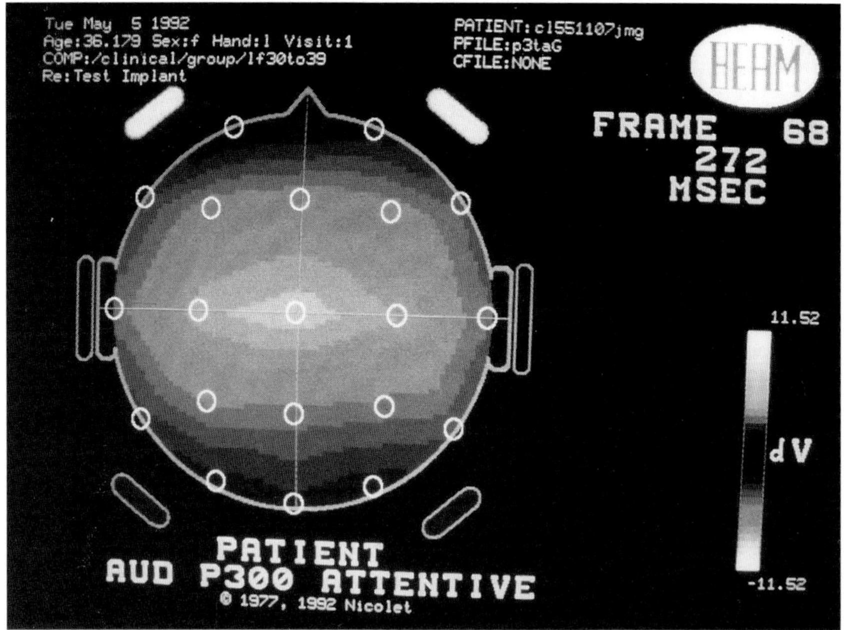

a

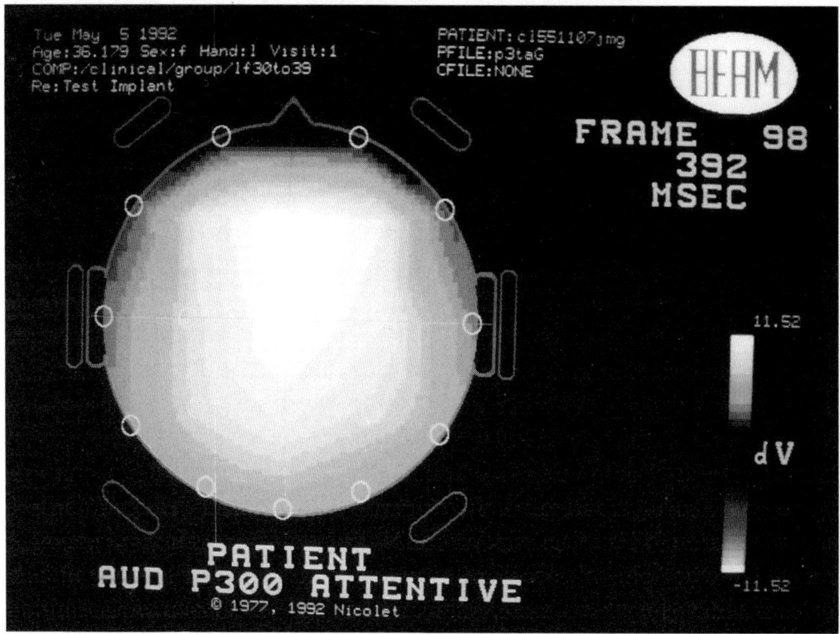

b

Fig. 5. Brain mapping. Cognitive evoked potentials. Same patient as in figure 3. *a* Mismatch negativity. *b* P 300.

In contrast, when for this same patient who, remember, is a star patient, we are studying the cognitive potentials, we find a perfectly well-defined P300 (fig. 4), in other words a cognitive capacity for excellent frequential discrimination.

The P300 appears perfectly normal, with excellent amplitude in the order of 11.5 μV. You can observe the mismatch negativity N200 that precedes the normal P300.

Note that the topography (fig. 5a, b) is more stereotyped and the curves show levels that are decidedly more marked than in the charting of late evoked auditory potentials. The amplitude is in the order of 11 μV, which is normal. It should be mentioned that the latencies of the appearance of the MMN and the P300 are indeed delated.

Conclusion

What is to be concluded from this preliminary work?

(1) By brain mapping, late auditory evoked potentials can be recorded at the level of the scalp, essentially contralaterally in wearers of a cochlear implant, who are stimulated acoustically via the speech processor of the implant.

These responses do not, however, correspond to the usual pattern, neither from the latency point of view nor from those of form or amplitude.

The responses originating from the auditory cortex of implanted patients, if they are present, cannot be compared with those of patients having normal hearing.

(2) The cognitive endogenous potentials can be recorded normally. This means that the cognitive capacities of frequential discrimination are excellent in certain patients, even should the pattern of late auditory evoked potentials not appear to be normal.

In other words, electric stimulation produced by the cochlear implant does stimulate the cortex, but in an abnormal manner. This information can nevertheless be of use to the implanted person who recognizes them and who finds a meaning in them, as shown by the cognitive endogenous potentials that may be perfectly normal.

We are proposing to continue this investigation in studying more closely the frequential discrimination capacities of implanted patients and also their frequential field.

This could perhaps enable the results of 'star patients' to be objectified.

At this stage of the study, however, given the artefacts of responses obtained by purely electric stimulations, brain mapping cannot yet be considered as an examination predictive of the quality of results to be obtained in the future implanted patient.

References

1 Guerit JM: Les potentiels évoqués. Masson, Paris, 1991, p 46.
2 Hopkins F, et al: Clinical value of topographic mapping and quantified neurophysiology. Arch Neurol 1989;46:1133–1136.
3 Scherg M, et al: Evoked dipole source potentials of the human auditory cortex. EEG Clin Neurophysiol 1986;65:344–360.
4 Scherg M, et al: A source analysis of the late human auditory evoked potentials. J Cogn Neurosci 1989;1:336–355.
5 Shallop JK, et al: Electrically evoked auditory brain stem responses and middle latency responses obtained from patients with the Nucleus multichannel cochlear implant. Ear Hear 1990;11:5–15.

Pr. M. Gersdorff, University of Louvain, Cliniques Universitaires St. Luc,
10, avenue Hippocrate, B–1200 Bruxelles (Belgium)

Fraysse B, Deguine O (eds): Cochlear Implants: New Perspectives.
Adv Otorhinolaryngol. Basel, Karger, 1993, vol 48, pp 44–48

Steady State Evoked Potentials: A New Tool for the Accurate Assessment of Hearing in Cochlear Implant Candidates

G. Rance[a], *F.W. Rickards*[b], *L.T. Cohen*[a], *M.J. Burton*[a], *G.M. Clark*

[a]Department of Otolaryngology, and [b]Deafness Studies Unit,
Institute of Education, University of Melbourne, Parkville, Australia

Precise determination of residual hearing in prospective cochlear implant candidates is essential. As the minimum age of implantation for young children has reduced, the use of objective measures of hearing has become more important. At the University of Melbourne Cochlear Implant Clinic, steady state evoked potential (SSEP) assessments are routinely carried out on all candidates under the age of 5 years using a microcomputer and custom-designed hardware in the manner described by Cohen et al. [1].

Steady state evoked potentials are scalp potentials elicited in response to sinusoidally amplitude and/or frequency modulated tones. The resulting potential is periodic, and is phase locked to the modulation envelope of the stimulus.

Good estimations of behavioural thresholds have been reported across a range of carrier frequencies (250–4,000 Hz), in both normal and hearing-impaired awake adults using SSEP testing techniques at repetition rates of 40 Hz [2, 3]. In addition to these findings, Cohen et al. [1] demonstrated that the response can be elicited by stimuli at low sound pressure levels in sleeping adults if modulation rates above 70 Hz are used. We have also successfully employed these high modulation frequencies to test sleeping neonates, obtaining results consistent with those seen in awake and sleeping adults, and suggesting that this technique is suitable for use as a measure of hearing acuity in sleeping children [4]. Furthermore, Rickards et al. [5] showed good agreement between SSEP thresholds and tone pip elicited

ABR thresholds to stimuli at 500 and 4,000 Hz, in a group of 20 neonates.

This paper presents the preliminary findings for a study examining the relationship between the SSEP thresholds observed in a group of young cochlear implant candidates, with thresholds obtained behaviourally. Data from a similar study involving hearing-impaired adults is also included.

Methods

Subjects in this study were 25 severely/profoundly hearing impaired children (12 male and 13 female). The median age of this group was 28 months with a range of 10–58 months at the time of the SSEP evaluation. In addition, the results of 35 adults (23 male and 12 female) with mild to severe degrees of hearing loss are also presented. None of the subjects showed any evidence of middle ear, and, in the case of the adults, retrocochlear dysfunction.

Subjects' hearing sensitivity was assessed behaviourally using a standard clinical procedure, with pure or warble tones and a clinical audiometer. Results were obtained in the free field or under headphones as dictated by the age of the child.

At the time of the SSEP data collection, the adults were in natural sleep, and the children were either sedated with chloralhydrate, or under a general anaesthetic. This assessment was typically carried out on the occasion of the child's CT scans.

Stimulus generation, recording procedures and waveform analysis were the same as described previously by Cohen et al. [1]. The presence or absence of a response was determined automatically using a detection criterion which looked for non-random phase behaviour in regular samples of the scalp potentials. The stimuli, presented via mu-metal screened TDH-39 headphones, were pure tones amplitude and frequency modulated at a rate of 90 Hz. Carrier frequencies from 250 Hz to 4,000 Hz were tested (typically in octave increments). The maximum sound levels of the stimuli were 104 dBHL for the 250-Hz carrier, and 120 dBHL for the 500-, 1,000-, 2,000- and 4,000-Hz carrier frequencies.

Results

Figure 1 shows the plot of SSEP thresholds (Y) versus clinical behavioural thresholds (X) obtained for all of the subjects using a 1-kHz stimulus together with the appropriate linear regression line. The slope of less than unity and positive intercept reflects the better threshold accuracy seen in ears with a greater degree of hearing loss. Regression lines drawn for other carrier frequencies followed a similar pattern.

A comparison of actual and predicted SSEP thresholds was carried out for each of the carrier frequencies. In 395 of the 412 comparisons (96%),

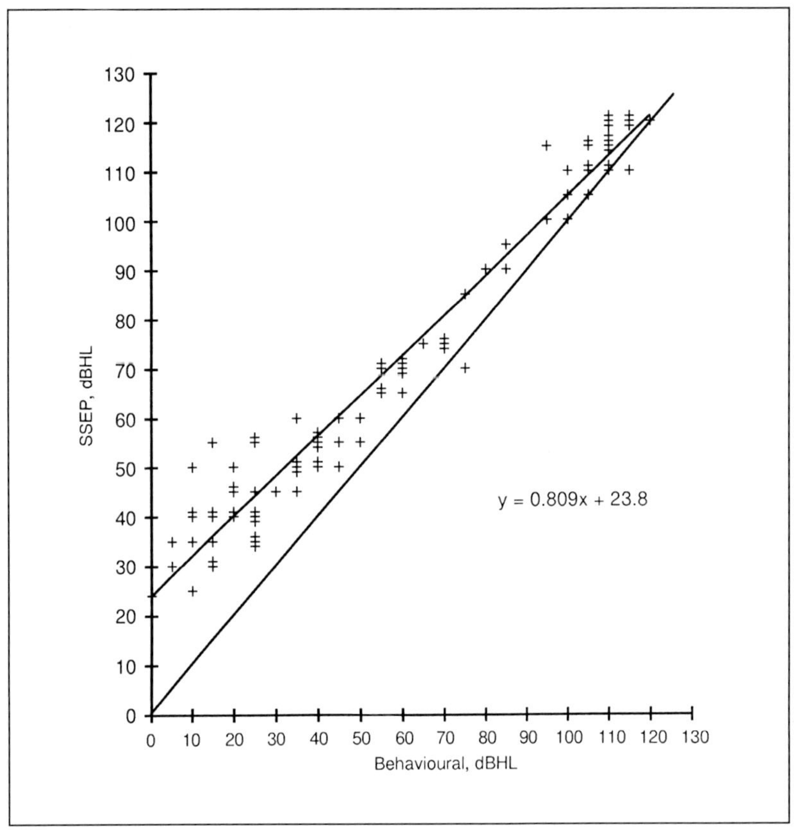

Fig. 1. Regression line analysis of threshold estimation using the SSEP technique in sleeping subjects to 1,000-Hz tones amplitude and frequency modulated at 90 Hz. Shown are the SSEP thresholds versus behavioural thresholds for 25 profoundly hearing impaired children, and 35 adults with mild to severe losses.

the observed SSEP threshold was found to be within 10 dB of that predicted by the regression line. Discrepancies of greater than 10 dB were only seen at the 250-, 500-, and 1,000-Hz carrier frequencies.

Of the 25 cochlear implant candidates included in this study, 14 showed only low frequency residual hearing (<1 kHz) when assessed behaviourally. SSEP testing carried out in the high frequencies on these subjects revealed no response to the stimuli at maximum levels indicating that artifactual responses were not contaminating the results.

In many cases the SSEP thresholds in the low frequencies were less than the behavioural thresholds in the octave frequency above, confirming that the responses to these frequency specific stimuli are likely to be originating from the appropriate place in the cochlea.

Discussion

The preliminary results presented in this paper suggest that a linear regression analysis can be used to predict behavioural thresholds from steady state evoked potential thresholds. Our data has shown that the use of the regression line will enable prediction of behavioural thresholds across a range of carrier frequencies, to within 10 dB accuracy on 96% of the occasions.

Threshold estimation using the SSEP technique, offers a number of advantages over other frequency specific evoked potential procedures in the assessment of young cochlear implant candidates. Middle latency and slow cortical responses for example, have been shown to be unreliable in young subjects due to maturational and sleeping effects.

Recent work using auditory brainstem responses to short duration tones in notched noise, has shown that threshold estimates in awake adult subjects can also be made with reasonable accuracy [6]. The evoked potential thresholds obtained from the normal and hearing impaired subjects in this paper were, however, more variable than those we obtained using the SSEP technique. Their results did show the improved accuracy with hearing impairment, and higher stimulus frequency seen in this study.

Another disadvantage of the ABR technique is that like all brief stimuli procedures, the equivalent dBHL levels at which it can test are limited. The continuous modulated tone used in the SSEP technique can be presented at levels as high as 120 dBHL, whereas click or brief tone stimuli are typically restricted to levels less than 100 dBnHL. This limitation is obviously a significant disadvantage when testing implant candidates with profound to total hearing losses.

Another advantage which the SSEP procedure has over transient evoked response techniques is that it does not require subjective waveform analysis. The periodicity of the potential allows automated response detection systems such as the one used in this study, to be employed. This approach may in part account for the small variability in threshold estimates that we have observed.

In summary, this test has shown a high degree of accuracy in the determination of hearing thresholds. The SSEP procedure is well suited as a measure of residual hearing in young cochlear implant candidates in that it can provide accurate thresholds to frequency-specific stimuli presented at high levels.

References

1 Cohen LT, Rickards FW, Clark GM: A comparison of steady-state evoked potentials to modulated tones in awake and sleeping humans. J Acoust Soc Am 1991;90:2467–2479.

2 Kuwada S, Batra R, Maher VL: Scalp potentials of normal and hearing impaired subjects in response to sinusoidally amplitude-modulated tones. Hear Res 1986;21: 179–192.

3 Stapells DR, Picton TW, Smith AD: Prediction of audiometric thresholds in normal and hearing impaired subjects using the 40Hz event related potential. Canadian Speech and Hearing Association Annual Convention, May 1983, Montreal.

4 Tan LE, Rickards FW, Cohen LT: Neonatal hearing screening using steady-state evoked potentials. Aust J Audiol 1988;(suppl 3).

5 Rickards FW, Wilson OJ, Tan LE, Cohen LT: Steady-state evoked potentials in normal neonates. Aust J Audiol 1990;(suppl 4):21.

6 Stapells DR, Picton TW, Durieux-Smith A, Edwards CG, Moran LM: Thresholds for short latency auditory evoked potentials to tones in notched noise in normal-hearing and hearing impaired subjects. Audiology 1990;29:262–274.

G. Rance, Department of Otolaryngology, University of Melbourne,
East Melbourne, Vic. 3002 (Australia)

Surgical Techniques

Fraysse B, Deguine O (eds): Cochlear Implants: New Perspectives.
Adv Otorhinolaryngol. Basel, Karger, 1993, vol 48, pp 49–58

Multichannel Implants in Postmeningitic Ossified Cochleas[1]

Simon C. Parisier, Patricia M. Chute

Cochlear Implant Center, Department of Otolaryngology, Head and Neck Surgery, Manhattan Eye, Ear and Throat Hospital, New York, N.Y., USA

Loss of hearing is a frequent complication of meningitis, having an incidence of between 8 and 24% [1, 2]. It is generally permanent, symmetrical, bilateral and, depending on the extent of injury, ranges from mild to profound. The infection from the brain-cerebrospinal fluid passes through the cribose areas of the internal auditory canal or the cochlear aqueduct and contaminates the inner ear fluids. The resulting labyrinthitis damages the organ of corti with loss of the hair cells. In addition, most cases develop labyrinthine neo-ossification (fig. 1) [3]. In the past 10 years, those unfortunate individuals who were so profoundly deafened that they were unable to benefit from amplification have had some degree of hearing restored by the electrical stimulation of auditory neurons using cochlear implants. The surgical insertion of these devices necessitates an open passageway through the scala tympani [4–7]. However, ossification of the cochlea may preclude the complete insertion of the cochlear-stimulating electrodes resulting in only a portion of the array being implanted (fig. 2).

This study reviews a series of 22 postmeningitic profoundly deaf children who had cochlear implants. The degree of cochlear ossification observed at surgery was compared with that detected on preoperative CT scans. The impact of ossification on the surgical insertion of the cochlear electrodes was analyzed. In cochleas that were obliterated by bone growth, the operative technique for inserting cochlear electrodes was reviewed.

[1] Funded by the Children's Hearing Institute.

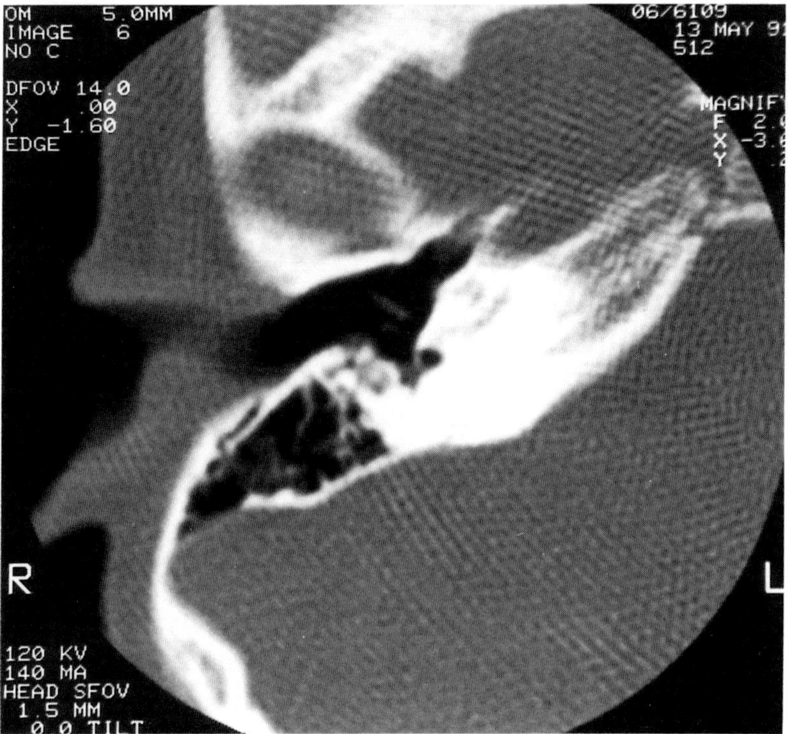

Fig. 1. Ossified cochlea postmeningitis. Fibrous bone occluding scala is less dense than the surrounding otic capsule.

The average number of electrodes that could be inserted was quantified and compared with the number that postoperatively could be electrically stimulated. The performance achieved with only a limited number of electrodes inserted was assessed and compared to those having had complete insertion.

Material and Methods

Material

The Cochlear Implant Center at Manhattan Eye, Ear and Throat Hospital in New York has performed cochlear implants on 85 patients using the 3M/House, 3M Vienna and the Cochlear Corporation's Nucleus 22 channel devices. The majority of patients have received the multi-channeled device which requires the insertion of an electrode

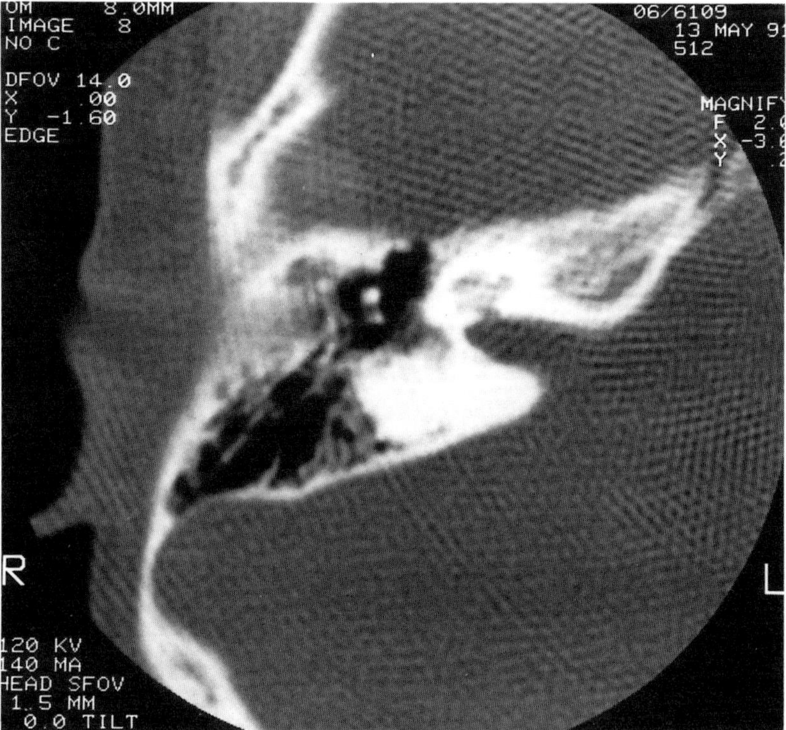

Fig. 2. Ossified lateral semicircular canal and cochlea postmeningitis.

array composed of 22 active stimulating platinum bands and 10 additional inactive retaining bands designed to facilitate its insertion into the cochlea.

Twenty-two children who became profoundly deaf after meningitis and received cochlear implants are the basis of this retrospective review. The infection was caused by *streptococcus pneumoniae* in 13 and by *Hemophilus influenza* in 9 patients. The age of the children at the time of surgery ranged from 2.5 to 17 years with 17 of the children under the age of 8 (average –7.6 years, median 5.6 years). The age at the time of the meningitis ranged from 9 months to 7 years with a mean of 2.9 years and a median of 2 years. The duration of deafness ranged from 6 months to 12 years, the average being 3.7 years and the median 2 years. The ratio of males to females was equal. Twenty of the children received Nucleus 22 channel cochlear implants and 2 the 3M/House device.

Methods

A retrospective review of the patient records was performed. A canal wall-up mastoidectomy with an extended facial recess approach allowed access to the middle ear space. The round window bony niche was drilled away to directly visualize the membrane. An opening into the cochlea was made anterior to the round window. The fenestra through which the electrode was inserted was made as anteriorly as was anatomically possible with the expectation that this would permit a more apical advancement of the electrode providing electrical stimulation to an area where there could be a larger number of surviving ganglion cells and nerve endings [1, 2].

Cochlear imaging was obtained preoperatively. A high-resolution scanner produced thin 1 mm axial and frequently coronal sections that provided sharply focused images of the cochleas and other structures within the temporal bones. Generally, these were performed without contrast. In younger children, sedation or general anesthesia was sometimes required. The CT scan and the operative reports of each subject were reviewed.

Based on the extent of cochlear ossification observed intraoperatively the children were placed into 1 of 5 categories: (classs 1) no ossification present; (class 2) round window membrane ossified; (class 3) ossification at the round window extending 0–2 mm into the scala tympani but coils patent; (class 4) ossification at the round window and 3–8 mm into the scala tympani but coils patent; (class 5) cochlea diffusely ossified with lumen obstruction.

The extent of ossification observed at surgery was compared with that reported on CT imaging.

Audiological test results included preoperative detection and perception data under headphones, with sensory aids (either amplication or with vibrotactile sensation). These same test results were obtained postoperatively, after cochlear implant.

Psychophysical test results obtained postoperatively were reviewed and included information regarding the number of electrodes that produced a response, the dynamic range of electrodes, the mode of stimulation and the encoding strategy utilized to generate the map.

Results

Characteristically, the neo-ossification that results after meningitis has a distinct appearance. It is chalky white and has a softer consistency than the cochlear capsule. In cases with incomplete bony obliteration drilling through this postinflammatory bone leads the surgeon to the fluid-filled scala. Ossification limited to the round window membrane and for a short distance within the scala tympani does not produce a significant barrier since it can easily be drilled away. However, as the basal turn of the cochlea is found to be more extensively ossified, the insertion of the electrode into a fluid-filled channel becomes progressively more challenging (fig. 3).

Twenty children were treated with multichannel cochlear implants, two with 3M/House single channel devices. In 3 cases (class 1) no neo-ossification had developed, the round window membrane was mobile and the scala tympani patent. CT scans had demonstrated normal cochleas.

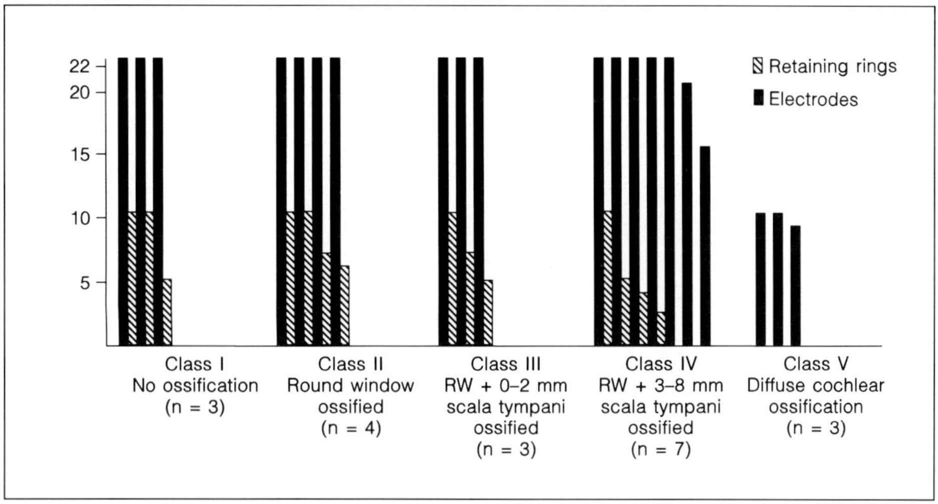

Fig. 3. Postmeningitis cochlear implant Nucleus 22/N-20 electrode, retaining rings insertion.

Four children were found to have isolated round window ossification (class 2). In these cases, a fenestration was made anterior to the round window to gain access to the fluid-filled scala tympani. Of these 4 children, only 1 was correctly diagnosed on CT scans.

Twelve children exhibited class 3 and 4 ossification, i.e. ossification from the round window extending 3–8 mm into the scala tympany. In these cases, it was possible to drill through the area of bone growth into an intact scala tympany. However, in 2 a limited number of electrodes, 15 and 20, could be inserted. Four of these 12 children were correctly identified preoperatively.

Finally, 3 children demonstrated complete cochlear ossification (class 5). These were correctly identified on preoperative CT scans. This occluding bone growth restricted the number of electrodes that could be implanted. Using an extended facial recess approach, drilling into the basal turn following the chalky white ossified plug as a guide, an 8–10 mm bony through that extended for the length of the basal portion of the cochlea was created. The length of the trough was limited by the coiling of the cochlea and its proximity to the carotid canal. Eight to 12 platinum bands could be placed within the drilled out bony channel. The electrode was immobilized by packing it into the surgically created defect using temporalis fascia.

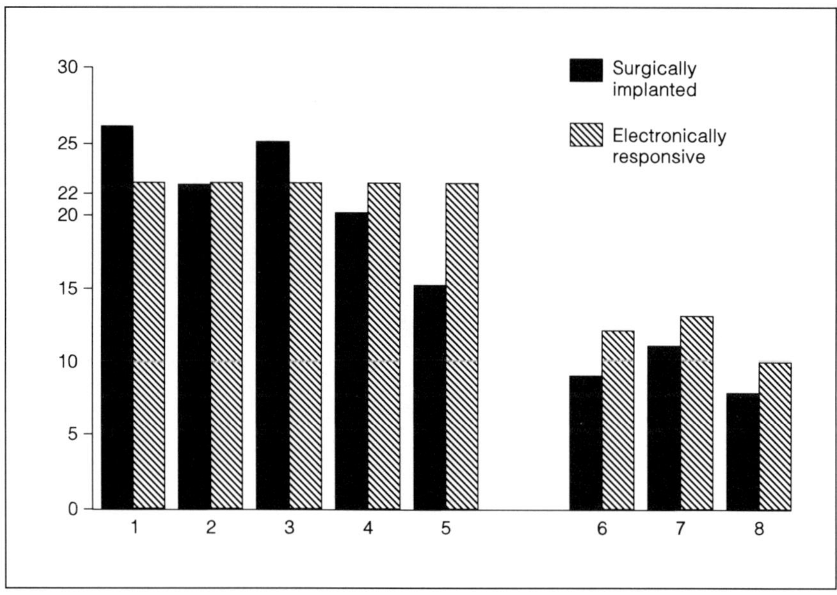

Fig. 4. Incomplete insertion retaining rings, electrodes correlation: surgically inserted electrodes vs. electrodes responding to electrical stimulation.

In summary, at surgery, no ossification – class 1 – was encountered in 3. The remaining patients all had bony cochlear involvement. A discretely ossified round window membrane – class 2 – was encountered in 4. Neo-ossification for 2 mm or less – class 3 – occurred in 5. Ossification extending 3–8 mm into the scala tympani – class 4 – in 7. Diffuse ossification of the cochlea – class 5 – in 3.

The accuracy of CT scans in these patients was assessed. CT scan imaging correctly demonstrated that in 3 cases no ossification was present. At the other extreme, 3 patients with extensive cochlear ossification were also correctly diagnosed radiographically. The remaining 16 children were found to have varying degrees of ossification at surgery but CT scans correctly identified the obstructing bone in only 5 patients. Overall, CT scanning was only 50% accurate in predicting the condition of the cochlea in children deafened from meningitis.

The first cochlear implant to be used in children was the 3M/House device. Three children initially received this single-channel cochlear im-

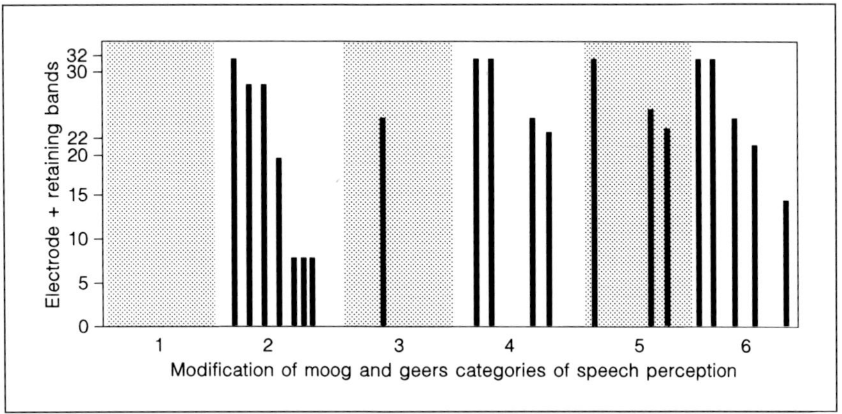

Fig. 5. Relationship between number of electrode and retaining bands inserted and category of speech perception achieved.

plant. In all 3 (2 in class 2, 1 in class 3) the 6-mm platinum electrode was entirely inserted in spite of some ossification. In 1 child, the device failed and was replaced with a Cochlear 22 channel implant.

Twenty of the children were implanted with the Nucleus 22 channel devices. Fifteen had all the active electrodes inserted. In 2 with class 3 and 4 type ossification, it was possible to insert only 15 and 21 electrodes, respectively, while in 3 children with class 5 ossification, only 9–12 electrodes could be inserted. The number of retaining rings that could be inserted in the 15 children who had all 22 electrodes inserted varied. All 10 retaining rings were inserted in 6, another had 5–9 retaining rings while 3 children with class 4 ossification had only 0–4 retaining rings inserted.

Postoperatively, the number of electrodes that responded to electrical stimulation was compared with the number reported to have been surgically implanted. A close correlation was observed (fig. 4). Frequently, the number of electrodes that produced an auditory sensation when electrically stimulated was slightly greater than that reported as having been surgically inserted.

The psychoacoustic performance of the 20 children with cochlear 22 implants (fig. 5) as classified using a modification of the Geers and Moog Categories of Speech Perception: (category 1) no pattern perception; (category 2) pattern perception; (category 3) some word recognition; (category

4) consistent word recognition; (category 5) some open set speech recognition; (category 6) consistent open set speech recognition. Categories 5 and 6 are additions to the traditional use of this classification system [8].

Seven children with full insertions had all 10 retaining rings inserted. They achieved category 6 in 2, category 5 in 1, category 4 in 2. The remaining child who was 4 years old and only 3 months postimplant had only reached category 2.

Six children who had 5–9 retaining rings inserted were classified as follows: 1 in category 6, 1 in category 5, 1 in category 4, 1 in category 3 and 3 in category 2. However, it must be noted that 1 of these in the last category is two and a half and has had the implant for only 6 months.

The 2 children with 0–4 retaining rings were classified into categories 6, 5 and 4, respectively.

Two children had partial insertions – 1 with 20 electrodes achieved category 2 and the other with 15 electrodes, category 6. The 3 remaining children with partial insertions into ossified cochleas are all classified as category 2 pattern perceivers. This is despite long-term use of the implant (2 years) and carefully monitored training.

Discussion

The labyrinthitis that occurs in children with meningitis is caused by the transmission of infected cerebrospinal fluid directly to the perilymphatic inner ear spaces and neo-ossification frequently develops within the membranous labyrinth. This post-inflammatory bone has a specific texture; it seems to be more fibrous and has a chalkier color than the adjacent normal labyrinthine capsule. One can speculate that if the contamination occurs through the cochlear aqueduct, the round window and contiguous scala tympany may discretely become ossified. These isolated areas of new bone growth may not be appreciated on CT scans which in these cases frequently were reported as being normal. However, if contamination occurs through the cribose areas within the porous area of the internal auditory canals, the contiguous semicircular canals and cochlea may become ossified producing a much more obvious CT image.

Localized areas of neo-ossification may not be radiographically imaged even with thinly sliced, properly positioned, high-definition CT scans because the postinflammatory bone may be less dense, more fibrous and may contain less calcium. Consequently, in children with profound hearing loss caused by meningitis, the otologist should expect to encounter some degree of ossification within the basal turn of the cochlea even when the CT scan is normal. Usually, the bone growth can be drilled through and the electrode placed within a fluid-filled cochlear coil. Thus, the neo-ossification of the cochlea after meningitis is not a contraindication for cochlear implant. In this report, the full 22 stimulating electrodes could be inserted in 12 of 14 children with ossification of the round window and/or scala tympani. In two others, 20 and 15 electrodes were inserted into an intact perilymphatic-filled scala tympani which had been accessed after drilling through significant ossification (class 4). One of 2 children with 15 electrodes has developed open set discrimination in spite of the reduced number of electrodes inserted. Thus, insertion of all electrodes and retaining rings is only one of many factors that determines how well a child will perform following a cochlear implant.

Three children had totally ossified cochleas: a 7-year-old with 5-years' duration of deafness, a 4 and a 5½ year old both of whom had been deaf for 2 years. They did not benefit to the same extent as most of the children in whom electrodes had been inserted into a perilymphatic fluid space. In order to reach auditory threshold with electrical stimulation, more power was required. Another factor that may restrict the auditory benefits of cochlear implants in children deafened from meningitis is a reduction in spiral ganglion cells that corresponds to areas of cochlear ossification. Those children with completely ossified cochleas would have a reduced number of spiral ganglion cells [1, 2].

The psychoacoustic development of these 3 children after implant was very slow and they were only able to attain category 2 (pattern perception) when classified using a modification of Geers and Moog categories of speech perception. However, they use their cochlear implants during their waking hours and benefit from auditory stimulation.

References

1 Nadol JB Jr: Hearing loss as a sequela of meningitis. Laryngoscope 1978;88:739–755.

2 Hinojosa R, Green DJ Jr, Marion MS: Ganglion cell population in labyrinthitis ossificans. Am J Otol 1991;12(suppl):3–7.

3 Eisenberg LS, Luxford WM, Becker TS, House WF: Electrical stimulation of the auditory system in children deafened by meningitis. Otolaryngol Head Neck Surg 1984;92:700–705.

4 Balkamy T, Gantz B, Nadol JB Jr: Multichannel cochlear implants in partially ossified cochleas. Ann Otol Rhinol Laryngol 1988;97(suppl 135):3–7.
5 Gantz BJ, McCabe BF, Tyler RS: Use of multichannel cochlear implants in obstructed and obliterated cochleas. Otolaryngol Head Neck Surg 1988;98:72–81.
6 Lambert PR, Ruth RA, Hodges AV: Multichannel cochlear implant and electrically evoked auditory brainstem responses in a child with labyrinthitis ossificans. Laryngoscope 1991;101:14–19.
7 Novak MA, Fifer RC, Barkmeier JC, Firszt MA: Labyrinthine ossification after meningitis: Its implications for cochlear implantation. Otolaryngol Head Neck Surg 1990;103:351–356.
8 Geers AE, Moog JS: Predicting spoken language acquisition of profoundly hearing-impaired children. J Speech Hear Disord 1987;52:84–94.

Simon C. Parisier, MD, 210 E. 64th Street, New York, NY 10021 (USA)

Fraysse B, Deguine O (eds): Cochlear Implants: New Perspectives.
Adv Otorhinolaryngol. Basel, Karger, 1993, vol 48, pp 59–61

Surgical Difficulties with Cochlear Implants

M. Portmann, D. Portmann, M. Négrevergne
Institut G. Portmann, Bordeaux, France

Cochlear implants surgery differs with the type of implant used. Extracochlear devices are easier to implant and surgery is advised for all causes of deafness. The device is placed outside the abnormal cochlea.

The better results achieved with multielectrode cochlear implants makes them preferable in all cases, but the pathology responsible for the deafness may make placing them difficult.

We chose three examples from the main groups of implants according to their placements.

Case Presentation

Post-traumatic deafness secondary to two fractures of the petrous bone. Meningitis infection in childhood with intracochlear ossification. Congenital cochlear malformation. The important malformations are clearly visible. Minor malformations can only be seen at operation. Our example is a microcochlea.

Results

We have always been successful in placing intracochlear implants but with some difficulty.

Initially, post-traumatic deafness was treated with a single-channel extracochlear electrode device. We were obliged to perform two operations to obtain good placement of the multi-channel intracochlear electrode. During the first operation the newly formed bone around the extracochlear electrode into the fracture under the basal turn of the cochlea. The control X-ray confirmed this and the second operation allowed us to place the electrode in the intracochlear position. The patient obtained a much better result than with the single-channel extracochlear electrode.

The second case is one of childhood meningitis with surgery being performed as an adult. Both cochlears seemed to be ossified on CT scan and we chose the best side even though we could not find any intracochlear lumen. After long and delicate drilling, a gutter at the site where the cochlea should be found allowed us to place the electrode. A piece of cortical bone was held to the bony promontory with biologic glue. During the trial, high-intensity stimulation together with very poor isolation of the electrode made us use this multi-channel electrode like a single-channel electrode. Hopefully, the transcutaneous plug will allow the use of equipment which is more powerful but cheaper.

The third case is a congenital cochlear malformation. Again our choice was made according to the preoperative CT scan in favor of the cochlea which was open widest. The very small mastoid of a young lady allows only a very narrow posterior tympanotomy. The facial nerve was skeletonised and a combined approach with an intrameatal flap was helpful for this difficult placement in a very small cochlea. At the start of stimulation, the facial nerve response made Dr. Dauman decide to isolate the first electrodes. The result was satisfactory, and the implant works like a multichannel electrode.

Conclusion

The examples emphasize the importance of excellent quality preoperative imaging. A CT scan and MRI well-focussed on the cochleae are essential. In spite of such imaging bad surprises are possible during operations. The use of an implant with a transcutaneous plug allows adaptation for using different types of external prostheses.

From the surgical point of view, we advise adherence to the classical approach (posterior tympanotomy and intrameatal access). It allows direct drilling of the bony promontory, if necessary, in difficult cases (microcochlea). Training and experience of operators in this type of surgery is essential.

A simple solution is to have a single-channel extracochlear electrode available which is always easy to place in the round window regardless of the state of the cochlea, however with less satisfying results for the patient.

References

1 Battmer RD, Laszig R, Lehnhardt E: Electrically elicited stapedius reflex in cochlear implant patients. Ear Hear 1990;11:370–374.
2 Clark GM, Blamey PJ, Brown AM et al: The University of Melbourne Nucleus multi-electrode cochlear implant. Adv Otorhinolaryngol 1987;38:1–181.
3 Cochen NL, Hoffman RA, Stroschein M: Medical or surgical complications related to the nucleus multichannel cochlear implant. Ann Otol Rhinol Laryngol 1988;97: 8–13.
4 Lehnhardt E: Cochlear Implant Mini System 22 zur Versorgung ertaubter Kleinkinder. HNO 1990;38:161–165.
5 Lehnhardt E, Hirshorn MS (eds): Cochlear Implant. Eine Hilfe für beidseitig Taube. Berlin, Springer, 1987.
6 Négrevergne M: Implants cochléaires, que choisir? Rev Laryngol 1991;112:347–348.
7 Balkany TJ (guest ed): The Otolaryngologic Clinics of North America: The Cochlear Implant. Philadelphia, Saunders, 1986, vol 19, p 2.
8 Clark GM, Tong YC, Patrick JF: Cochlear Prostheses. Edinburgh, Churchill Livingstone, 1990.

Dr. M. Portmann, Institut G. Portmann, 114, avenue d'Arès,
F-33074 Bordeaux (France)

Fraysse B, Deguine O (eds): Cochlear Implants: New Perspectives.
Adv Otorhinolaryngol. Basel, Karger, 1993, vol 48, pp 62–64

Intracochlear Electrode Placement Facilitated by Healon®

E. Lehnhardt

Hals-Nasen-Ohrenklinik der Medizinischen Hochschule Hannover, BRD

In the cochlear implant operations we attempt, with the greatest of caution, to insert an electrode array as far as possible into the scala tympani because, even in deaf individuals, we assume that in the middle and upper turns we are more likely to find residual active hair cells and neural elements. The deep intracochlear placement of electrodes is only possible when the electrode carrier possesses optimal mechanical properties.

The flexibility of the Nucleus array is essential to allow the placement of the electrodes within the cochlea over a distance of 17 mm and, for example, within the frequency range between 5,000 and 1,000 Hz.

The experienced surgeon will have no difficulty inserting the Nucleus electrode carrier into an open lumen if it is free of fibrous tissue and filled with fluid. Indeed, one is always impressed by the ease with which the electrodes 'disappear' into the scala tympani. It is important, however, to make the insertion freely through the cochleostomy or the enlarged round window. The electrode carrier should not be pushed in with alligator forceps but rather with the claws supplied in the Nucleus surgical kit. This must be done very delicately. If resistance is encountered, it is possible to attempt to continue insertion by carefully turning the implant in the direction of the turn of the cochlea: counter-clockwise in the right ear and clockwise in the left.

Except for the disappointing situation for both patient and doctor in which a cochlea is partially or mostly obliterated, we can often insert all rings, even some blind rings, up to the cochleotomy. The question has arisen, however, as to what we can do for the more difficult cases – whether or not it is possible to insert the electrode array even further into the

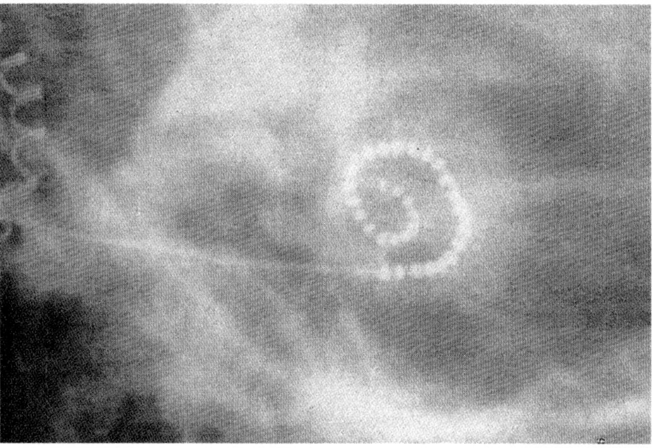

Fig. 1. Plane X-ray view on 17.01.92 with the electrode carrier reaching the apical half of the medial turn.

cochlea. To facilitate this, the lubricant Healon, a hyaluronic acid, was chosen [1]. It is made of an extract from a cock's comb and is, therefore, of biological origin. Hyaluronic acid is available in the form of a visco-elastic gel (Healon®, Pharmacia AB, Uppsala, Sweden) and is mostly used in ophthalmology when extracting the human lens in order to maintain the volume of the anterior chamber. In addition, it serves to protect the endothelium of the anterior chamber during surgical procedures. It is also used to coat intraocular lenses. Due to its high molecular weight (5 million), it has specific viscosity and is thus recommended as a 'visco-surgical' instrument.

Hyaluronic acid is found – in animals and humans – in the extracellular matrix of the connective tissue, in the synovial fluid, in skin and also in the vitreous body and in the chamber fluid of the eye. Hyaluronic acid has no ototoxic effect, even when used in high concentrations. According to current knowledge, clinical use of hyaluronic acid appears to be safe.

In utilising Healon in cochlear implant surgery, we hoped for easier insertion of the electrode carrier as it travels along the walls of the scala tympani and also to achieve a protective effect for the fibrous layer, especially along the lateral wall and the spiral ligament.

To achieve this, we pulled the electrode carrier through a drop of hyaluronic acid just before inserting it into the opened cochlea, and also

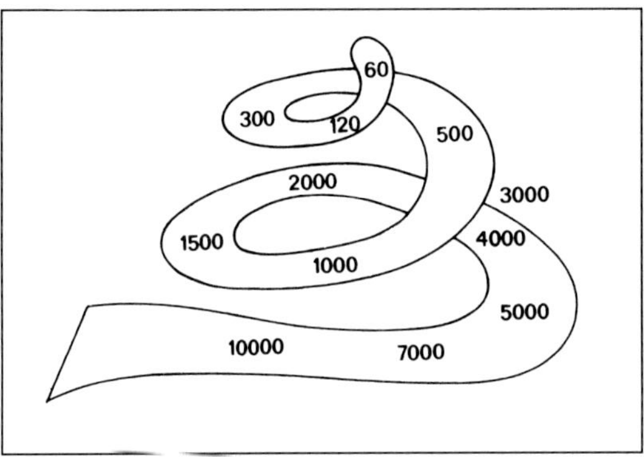

Fig. 2. Tonotopy of the human cochlea.

applied a second drop through a very soft silastic tube into the scala tympani. The advantage of increasing the ease of insertion by lubricating the electrode array was apparent. Even the blind rings often disappeared into the cochlea as long as there was an unobstructed lumen. In the optimal case, even the apical half of the middle turn can be reached without force (fig. 1). This more apical location correlates to the frequency region of approximately 4,000 to 400 Hz as compared to the usual location of 5,000 to 1,000 Hz (fig. 2).

Careful analysis of functional results will show what practical uses can result from this modification in the insertion technique.

Reference

1 Minisymposium on 'Hyaluronan and Its Use in Clinical Otology', Uppsala, 1986. Acta Otolaryngol (Stockh) 1986;(suppl 442):1–94.

Prof. E. Lehnhardt, Siegesstrasse 15, D–30175 Hannover (FRG)

Fraysse B, Deguine O (eds): Cochlear Implants: New Perspectives.
Adv Otorhinolaryngol. Basel, Karger, 1993, vol 48, pp 65–69

Problems in Cochlear Implant Surgery

Gregorio Babighian

Department of Otolaryngology, Ospedali Civili Riuniti, Venice, Italy

The standardisation of the surgical procedure for the intracochlear implantation of an electronic device in the totally deaf ear relies upon three technical keypoints: (1) the introduction along the scala tympani of an electrode array and its stabilisation; (2) the creation of a seat for the internal receiver/stimulator into the squama temporalis, and (3) the elevation of a wide, well vascularized skin flap, adequate to cover without tension the internal package of the implanted device [1–4]. With all the devices, the electrode is inserted into the cochlea via an opening at or near the round window, and the approach to the latter requires a Canal Wall Up procedure, with a limited mastoidectomy and a deep posterior tympanotomy, in order to expose widely the facial recess.

When the above mentioned points are skillfully realized in well-selected candidates, unwanted drawbacks seldom occur. Actually, major complications, i.e. requiring revision surgery do not exceed 5% of cases [5], however, some problems can be unexpectedly encountered, demanding for specific technical solutions. Among these, the following will be here considered: (1) Delayed wound breakdown. (2) Chronic otitis. (3) Cochlear obliteration.

Methods

One case out of 30 occurred in our case material with the partial exposure of the antenna of the receiver-stimulator about 1 month postoperatively. The complication was successfully managed through the excision of an ellypse of skin including the devitalized areas with wide healthy borders. The electronic package was left untouched, the fresh borders were mobilized and layer-sutured. The patient is consequently using her device for the entire waketime since 1 year.

Some cases are more difficult to be treated, for instance in case of an active infection, and the explantation is advisable, with the reimplantation to be performed at a later date [6]. There may also be the need to raised local flaps, but in some instances it is sufficient to perform an additional skin incision, prolonging the original one to the temporoparietal area. The internal package is then gently lifted out from its bed and transposed superior to the auricle. The mastoid area and the electrode array are left undisturbed [7]. This technique can be adopted in the case of either a former postauricular C incision (often associated with flap breakdown cases) or an inverted U or an extended endaural flap (the most safe in this regard).

Should the electrode array be explanted, surgical maneuvers must be very gentle and if reimplantation is foreseen it is advisable to leave intracochlear the tip of the electrode in order to secure the permeability of the track until the repositioning of a new device.

Cochlear implantation in chronic otitis media and its sequelae is performed, in general, as a planned second stage surgery.

This holds true, in our hands, even in case of a simple tympanic perforation without infection. Myringoplasty, either underlay or overlay, is performed as the first stage procedure, the cochlear implantation ensues 3–4 months later.

In 2 cases we had to revise a former Canal Wall Up tympanoplasty procedure, with a wide tympanic membrane perforation and a deep sinus tympani.

The tympanoplasty was revised as usually: the mastoid cavity was cleaned and shaped following the usual anatomic landmarks; the posterior tympanotomy was deepened, the tympanic membrane was repaired. Then, in order to obtain a wider exposure of the sinus tympani, the posterior bony wall was temporarily removed using a Feldmann saw. After exploration and cleaning of the involved area, the wall was repositioned and cemented to its bony borders by means of an ionomeric cement. The 2nd operation was carried out 3 and 5 months later, respectively.

When the device has to be implanted in an open cavity, the available options to the surgeon are the repair of the posterior wall, using, for instance, the Magnan hydroxyapatite posterior wall; or the partial obliteration of the cavity and the insertion of the electrode array beneath the flap covering the cavity itself [8].

In an old radical cavity, we partially obliterated the cavity, using hydroxyapatite granules mixed with autogenous bone paté. The mucosa was removed and the tubal opening obliterated with a cartilagineous plug. The external auditory meatus was sealed with an everting suture. The promontorium as well as the obliterating material were covered with a fascial flap. Subsequently, a wide temporalis muscle pedicled flap was laid down into the cavity. The postoperative course was uneventful. Six months later the 2nd stage operation was performed. The tympanomastoid plug was elevated and the electrode array was positioned down to the mastoid bony wall and over the flattened fallopian bridge. Then it was inserted through the cochleotomy, into the cochlea. The array having shown too long, it was partially wrapped up and sealed into the antral cavity, out of the middle ear cleft, by means of a small amount of ionomeric cement.

Bony or fibrous obliteration of the cochlea is a major issue for the surgeon [9, 10]. Labyrinthitis ossificans is most frequently associated with meningitis with pneumococcal aetiology. Children having suffered from this disease show the largest ossification specially at the scala tympani (34%) and at the round window (50%) [11]. Tympanogenic meningitis is generally associated with complete ossification of the scala tympani, whereas in labyrinthine otosclerosis the ossification is usually limited to the first few millimeters proximal to the round window.

By no means is cochlear ossification an absolute contraindication to cochlear implantation. Cochlear patency must be assessed preoperatively by means of modern imaging techniques [12, 13]. CT is a reliable predictor of partial or total ossification when resulting abnormal. In fact, in case of a normal CT, false-negative responses occur in 46% of the cases [12], due to the lesions being beyond the resolution power of the CT, or to low-density lesions, irregularly spread along the cochlear turns [14].

MRI is particularly useful for evidencing the membranous labyrinth: fibrosis, limited ossification or changes progressing to ossification can be detected [15].

Techniques for the management of the patient with an ossified cochlea differ according to the extension of the obliteration.

If ossification is strictly limited to the round window and the first 3–4 mm of the scala tympani, conventional drilling is performed anterioinferior to round window caring not to enter a deep hypotimpanic cell. In most cases, removal of the whitish newly formed bone with a very small diamond bur and under irrigation for 3–5 mm will lead to the lumen of the scala tympani.

In case of a more extended ossification the electrode can be introduced into the scala vestibuli through the oval window [16], or the cochlear labyrinth can be exenterated into the middle ear, and the electrode laid down into the bony gutter such obtained [17].

This technique normally requires a wide acces to the middle ear through a radical mastoidectomy, the removal of the middle ear mucosa and the obstruction of the tubal opening. The cochlear labyrinth is drilled open close to the labyrinthine segment of the facial nerve and the internal carotid artery. The electrode array is positioned, as said, into the gutter and sealed in place with a temporalis fascia flap.

We performed this procedure in two cases. The most important landmark is provided by the very sharp boundary line between the yellowish bone of the otic capsule and the white new bone. This line guides the drilling along the different segments of the basal turn up to the middle turn and even close to the apex. The facial nerve function is constantly monitored intraoperatively.

If the ossification does not involve more than the basal turn then we advise to avoid a radical mastoidectomy technique. Instead, a Canal Wall Up operation is performed and using a Feldmann saw the posterior bony canal wall is cut and displaced anteriorly. The basal turn is drilled along the above-mentioned boundary line until the lumen of the scala tympani is found. The electrode array is then inserted and sealed in place using a few fascial pledgets soaked with fibrin sealant.

Conclusions

Major complications requiring revision surgery and specially related to the implantation of a cochlear electronic device are rather uncommon [6] and do not exceed, an average, 5% of the cases. Minor complications, resolving spontaneously or requiring minimal treatment, occur in about

7% of the cases [5]. In our still limited experience (30 postlingual patients) complications requiring revision surgery occurred in 2 cases (6.6%). More frequent are those pathological conditions requiring a specific technical solution from the surgeon ossification of the labyrinth or sequelae of surgey for chronic otitis media with or without cholesteatoma are two significant examples of such adverse conditions.

The relatively limited case material of the large majority of surgeons dealing with cochlear implantation involves, as a consequence, that the procedures reported here have been performed in a rather low number of patients. Nonetheless, these procedures seem to offer valuable and proven solutions to the problems which are likely to affect or even to hinder a cochlear implantation. More well-documented reports will probably confirm these preliminary successful achievements.

References

1 Luxford WM, House WF: House 3M cochlear implant: Surgical considerations. Ann Otol Rhinol Laryngol 1987;(suppl 128)96:12–14.

2 Burian K, Hochmayr-Desoyer IJ, Eisenwort B: The Vienna cochlear implant program. Otolaryngol Clin North Am 1986;19:313–328.

3 Clark GM, Pyman BC, Webb RL, Bailey QE: The surgery for multiple electrode cochlear implantation. J Laryngol Otol 1979;93:215–223.

4 Clark GM, Pyman BC, Webb RL, Bailey QE, Shepherd RK: Surgery for an improved multiple channel implant. Ann Otol Rhinol Laryngol 1984;93:204–207.

5 Cohen NL, Hoffmann RA, Stroschein M: Medical or surgical complications related to the Nucleus multichannel cochlear implant. Ann Otol Rhinol Laryngol 1988;(suppl 135)97:8–13.

6 Webb, RL, Lehnhardt E, Clark GM, Laszig R, Pyman BC, Frank BK: Surgical complications with the Cochlear multiple-channel cochlear implant: Experience at Hannover and Melbourne. Ann Otol Rhinol Laryngol 1991;100:131–136.

7 Haberkamp TJ, Schwaber MK: Management of flap necrosis in cochlear implantation. Ann Otol Rhinol 1992;101:38–41.

8 Schloendorff G, Hermes H, Weck L: Cochlear implants in patients with radical cavity. HNO 1989;37:423–425.

9 Balkany T, Gantz B, Nadol JBjr: Multichannel cochlear implants in partially ossified cochleas. Ann Otol Rhinol Laryngol 1988;(suppl 135)97:3–7.

10 Green JDjr, Marion MS, Hinojosa R: Labyrinthitis ossificans: Histopathologic considerations for cochlear implantation. Otolaryngol Head Neck Surg 1991;104:320–326.

11 Luxford WM, House WF: Cochlear implants in children: Medical and surgical considerations. Ear Hear 1985;(suppl 3)6:20–23.

12 Jackler RK, Luxford WM, Schindler RA, McKerrow WS: Cochlear patency problems in cochlear implantation. Laryngoscope 1987;97:801–805.

13 Harnsberger HR, Dart DJ, Parkin JL, Smoker WR: Cochlear implant candidates: assessment with CT and MRI imaging. Radiology 1987;164:53–57.
14 Furia F, Fraysse B, Vandeventer G, Bonafe A, Berry I, Manelfe C: Imaging evaluation of cochlear implantation; in Fraysse B, Cochard N (eds): Cochlear Implant Acquisition and Controverses. Toulouse 1990, pp 165–168.
15 Yune HY, Miyamoto RT, Yune ME: Medical imaging in cochlear implant candidates. Am J Otol 1991;12:11–17.
16 Steenerson RL, Gary LB, Wynens MS: Scala vestibuli cochlear implantation for labyrinthine ossification. Am J Otol 1990;11:360–363.
17 Gantz BJ, McCabe BF, Tyler RS: Use of multichannel cochlear implants in obstructed and obliterated cochleas Otolaryngol Head Neck Surg 1988;98:72–81.

Prof. Dr. Gregorio Babighian, Dorsoduro 1023, I–30123 Venice (Italy)

Technical Failures

Fraysse B, Deguine O (eds): Cochlear Implants: New Perspectives.
Adv Otorhinolaryngol. Basel, Karger, 1993, vol 48, pp 70–74

Surgical Complications of Multichannel Cochlear Implants in North America

Noel L. Cohen, Ronald A. Hoffman

Department of Otolaryngology, NYU School of Medicine, New York, N.Y., USA

The complications of cochlear implant surgery are a reflection of the complexity of the surgical procedure, the skill of the operating surgeon and the risks inherent in the insertion of a large foreign body immediately deep to the scalp. As may be expected, those parts of the operation which are least commonly performed tend to have the highest rate of complication: creating a large scalp flap, approaching the middle ear via the facial recess, and inserting a flexible electrode array into the scala tympani via a cochleostomy.

Table 1 summarizes the complications which have occurred in 2,751 operations involving the Nucleus 22 channel device. Table 2 summarizes the complications resulting from 157 patients who have received the Ineraid Device. There are only two reported life-threatening complications in this entire group, both of them in patients who had meningitis associated with a CSF gusher. Both were treated and resolved completely.

Nucleus Device

Flap-related problems constitute the largest category of major and minor complications with the Nucleus implant. As expected, electrode placement was another of the more common areas of complications, while a number of patients suffered VIIth nerve paralysis at the time of or shortly following surgery.

Extrusion of the receiver/stimulator, migration of either electrodes or the receiver/stimulator, and device failures may not be related to surgical problems as much as to the device itself.

Table 1 lists the Nucleus flap-related problems in 1,995 adults and 756 children. An excessively thin flap is more likely to break down, especially when subjected to pressure by opposing magnets. Delayed flap healing and necrosis may be related to improper handling of the flap during surgery. The flap must be manipulated delicately, must not be allowed to dry during the surgery, and hemostasis must be meticulous. The first evidence of

Table 1. Nucleus (n = 2,751)

Major	Minor
2 meningitis	57 VII stimulation
63 flap	20 flap
52 device failure	16 electrode migration
48 electrode placement	9 dizzy
31 R/S migration/extrusion	7 tinnitus
20 VII palsy	4 electrode placement
4 other	1 R/S migration
220 (7.99%)	119 (4.33%)

Table 2. Ineraid (n = 157)

	17 major (= 10.83%), %
13 infection	8.3
6 infection with Re-op	3.8
2 electrode failure	1.3
3 sheared pedestal	1.9
9 explant	5.7
6 infection	3.8
3 trauma	1.9
2 hypotympanic electrode	1.3
4 flap problems, major	2.5
39	

flap infection or necrosis should be treated intensively in an attempt to avoid progression and potential loss of the device. Early culture and sensitivity should be followed by topical and oral antibiotics. If resolution is not prompt, hospitalization, intravenous antibiotics and more aggressive surgical management may be appropriate.

Facial Nerve Injury

The facial recess approach to the posterior mesotympanum places the facial nerve at risk. Moreover, particularly in children with congenital cochlear malformations, an anomalous facial nerve may be injured even by an experienced surgeon. Facial nerve injury may be minimized by using a facial nerve monitor, but even this is not a guarantee of avoidance of injury, either early or delayed.

Electrode Placement

A third area of common complication is electrode placement. Insertion must be very gentle, and pressure should never be exerted. An intraoperative X-ray in the operating room is strongly advised to confirm proper placement of the electrode, as well as the absence of kinking or compression.

Perilymph Gusher

Perilymph gusher should be anticipated when operating on a patient with an anomalous cochlea or a short/wide internal auditory canal. A gusher can usually be controlled by waiting for the flow of cerebrospinal fluid to abate and then firmly packing the cochleostomy with soft tissue. Continuous lumbar cerebrospinal fluid drainage may be a useful adjunct.

Postoperative Tinnitus and Dizziness

Postoperative tinnitus and dizziness are uncommon. Many implanted patients state that their tinnitus abates with the use of their implants. Dizziness may also occur postoperatively, and may require re-exploration for a perilymph fistula.

R/S Migration or Extrusion

Occasionally, the receiver/stimulator may migrate under the scalp flap. This should be minimal if the case is tied down to the side of the skull.

Receiver stimulator extrusion, on the other hand, may have to do with flap necrosis, excessive magnet force, or rarely an ideopathic reaction whereby the receiver stimulator extrudes through the scalp years following the surgery, in the absence of any infection or trauma. The mechanism of this delayed extrusion is unknown.

Device Failure

Although technically not a surgical complication, failure of the internal device requires re-operation in order to provide the patient with a functioning implant. This has occurred 52 times in 2,858 cases.

Ineraid Multichannel Cochlear Implant

The Ineraid device manufactured by Smith & Nephew Richards, is a multichannel device characterized by six intracochlear electrodes and a percutaneous pedestal (table 2). Most complications with this device are pedestal related. Thirteen cases required more than topical treatment. Six cases required explanation of the device because of infection.

Three patients required a new device because of fracture of the pedestal from external trauma. Four patients required revision flap surgery and two hypotympanic electrodes were reported. Two electrode failures also occurred. There have been no reported facial nerve problems or compressed electrodes with this device.

Table 3. Nucleus adult vs. child complications

	Adult (n = 1,995), %	Child (n = 756), %
Life threatening	0.1	0
Flap	3.46	1.85
VII palsy	0.65	0.93
Hypotympanic electrode	0.80	0.79
Compressed/kinked electrode	0.85	0.3
Delayed electrode migration	1.00	0.53
Gusher	0.05	0.53
R/S migration	0.20	0.13
R/S extrusion	1.30	0.13
Device failure (Mini 22)	1.08	1.81

Complications in Children

Due to the smaller size of the head, and the fact that the identical device is used for both adults and children, an increased number of complications might be anticipated in children, especially in the younger age group. In fact, there have been fewer complications overall in children than in adults. There has been no increased incidence of otitis media in the ears of children having a cochlear implant, and no complications when otitis media occurred in the presence of this large foreign body (table 3).

Summary

By paying careful attention to the details of surgical technique, many of the complications which have occurred to date may be avoided. Some, such as late electrode and receiver/stimulator migration, device failures, and late flap necrosis due to excessive magnetic forces cannot be avoided by the surgeon, but may be prevented by further advances in implant designs. Although the incidence of life-threatening complications is minimal, and that of major complications is acceptable, every effort should be made by the surgeon, audiologist and manufacturer to further diminish these problems.

Noel L. Cohen, MD, NYU School of Medicine, 550 First Avenue,
New York, NY 10016 (USA)

Fraysse B, Deguine O (eds): Cochlear Implants: New Perspectives.
Adv Otorhinolaryngol. Basel, Karger, 1993, vol 48, pp 75–78

Implant Generated Surface Potentials and (Partial) Device Failures of the Nucleus Cochlear Implant

Lucas H.M. Mens[a], *Thom Oostendorp*[b], *Paul van den Broek*[a, 1]

[a]University Hospital Nijmegen St. Radboud, and
[b]Department of Biophysics, University of Nijmegen, The Netherlands

At the moment there is no reliable way to test the integrity of multichannel implant devices such as the Nucleus system which lack a telemetric feedback option. In this paper an objective measurement technique is described with which a nonintermittent (partial) failure of the implant, including the electrode array, can be detected.

Surfaces potentials have been used in the past to discriminate between hardware problems and 'patient problems': for instance a child that cannot respond or perhaps refuses to respond. However, when recording surface potentials from a Nucleus implant operating in the normal Bipolar + 1 mode, in general very small amplitudes are found from the most apical electrodes. These small amplitudes, caused by the density of the cochlear bone, have erroneously been interpreted as a device malfunction.

Reliable surface recordings can be made a special stimulation strategy described in the following.

Method

In the Bipolar + 1 stimulation mode normally used for the Nucleus device, each of the 22 electrodes is used in combination with only one other electrode (e.g. 1 and 3, 2 and 4, etc.). A custom software package (MINT) from Cochlear AG allows stimulation on all

[1] The authors wish to thank Ernst von Wallenberg from Cochlear AG for his support. Teun Spies stimulated earlier steps towards this research. John Noten is acknowledged for his helping hand in electronics.

paired combinations of electrodes. For instance, electrode 1 is not only used in combination with electrode 2 or 3, but also in combination with electrode 4, 5, etc. up to 22. Of each pair, the most basal electrode is called the 'active electrode' and the most apical one the 'reference electrode'. For 21 active electrodes, 231 of such paired combinations can be made.

All stimuli were presented at the same stimulus amplitude: device-specific current level 50. A fixed pulse width of 200 μs was used.

Recordings were made between a surface electrode on the mastoid at the side of the implant and the forehead ('ipsilateral' recordings), or between the electrode on the mastoid at the side of the implant and an electrode on the contralateral mastoid ('bilateral' recordings).

A simple low-pass filter (cut-off frequency at 350 kHz) is inserted in the measurement leads [cf. 1]. It prevents saturation of the amplifier by the radiofrequency signal emitted by the transmitter.

The peak-to-peak amplitude of the averaged recordings is measured. Adopting a convention proposed by Heller et al. [2], negative-leading recorded waveforms are assigned a positive peak-to-peak amplitude.

Results

In table 1, the peak-to-peak amplitudes of all 231 recorded waveforms from subject 1 are given. Subject 1 had an intact electrode array. All waveforms were of the same phase (negative leading). The recordings from the apical electrode combinations did not rise above the background noise and are deleted from the table.

One marked advantage of the present stimulation strategy is that very clear recordings can be made from stimulation on electrode pairs that include the most apical electrodes, namely, in combination with basal active electrodes.

Overall, the recorded amplitude increased with distance between active and reference electrode along the basilar membrane, and decreased with distance from the round window.

In table 2 the peak-to-peak amplitudes are given of a recording from a patient with known failure in the electrode array. Surgical insertion of the electrode array was difficult and the array may well have been overstressed. The amplitudes on active electrode 3 are lower, and on active electrode 12 higher than on adjacent electrodes. On reference electrodes 12 and 20 relatively low amplitudes are measured; in combination with more apical electrodes, negative amplitudes (that is, phase reversals) are obtained. These indications of hardware problems on electrodes 12 and 20 are in agreement with an expert analysis of the behavioral threshold and

Table 1. Peak-to-peak amplitudes of surface potentials from patient 1

Active electrode																Reference electrode
16	15	14	13	12	11	10	9	8	7	6	5	4	3	2	1	
·	1	1	1	1	2	2	3	3	4	5	5	7	8	10	11	22
·	·	1	1	1	2	2	3	3	4	5	5	7	8	9	12	21
·	·	1	1	2	2	2	3	3	4	5	6	7	8	9	11	20
·	·	1	1	1	2	2	3	3	4	5	5	7	8	9	12	19
·	·	·	1	1	2	2	3	3	4	5	5	6	8	9	11	18
·	·	·	1	1	2	2	2	3	4	5	5	7	8	9	11	17
	·	·	1	1	1	2	2	3	3	4	5	6	7	8	11	16
		·	·	1	1	2	2	3	3	4	4	6	7	8	11	15
			·	1	1	1	2	2	3	4	5	6	7	8	10	14
				·	1	1	1	2	3	4	4	5	7	8	10	13
					·	1	1	2	2	3	4	5	6	8	10	12
						·	1	1	2	3	4	5	6	7	9	11
							·	1	2	2	3	4	5	6	8	10
								·	1	2	3	4	5	5	6	9
									·	1	2	4	4	6	8	8
										1	2	3	4	5	7	7
											1	2	3	4	7	6
												1	2	3	6	5
													1	3	5	4
														1	4	3
															3	2

Values are microvolts. Negative amplitudes are positive-leading waveforms. Recordings from active electrode 16 to 22 did not rise above the background noise (15–22 in table 2), as did the recordings indicated with a '·'.

comfort levels from this adult patient. Electrodes 1–6 are not used because these are outside the cochlea.

In sum, the recording of surface potentials using the stimulation strategy described above provides a useful means to check for complete or partial device failures. Especially in children, accurate threshold and comfort levels may not be available and an objective technique is required. It takes about 30 min and testing can be done at sub-threshold stimulus levels.

It has to be stressed that certain types of malfunctioning of the electrode array may not be detectable with the method described in this paper.

Table 2. Peak-to-peak amplitudes of surface potentials from patient 2

Active electrode																Reference electrode
16	15	14	13	12	11	10	9	8	7	6	5	4	3	2	1	
·	·	·	·	7	2	2	3	5	6	8	10	11	5	15	27	22
·	·	·	·	6	2	2	3	4	6	8	9	10	7	15	18	21
·	·	·	1	5	0	−1	2	3	4	6	7	8	4	12	14	20
·	·	·	1	6	2	2	3	4	6	8	9	10	6	15	17	19
·	·	·	1	7	2	2	3	4	6	8	9	10	7	14	18	18
·	·	·	−1	6	1	2	2	3	5	7	9	10	6	14	17	17
	·	−1	−1	6	1	2	2	3	5	7	8	9	6	14	17	16
		−1	−1	5	1	1	2	3	5	7	8	9	6	13	17	15
			−1	5	1	1	2	3	5	7	8	9	5	13	17	14
				5	0	1	2	3	4	7	7	8	5	13	16	13
					−5	−4	−3	−2	−1	1	3	4	3	8	11	12
						0	1	2	4	6	7	7	5	12	15	11
							0	1	3	5	6	8	4	12	15	10
								1	2	5	6	6	3	12	14	9
									2	4	5	6	2	10	13	8
										2	3	5	1	1	11	7
											2	2	−1	7	9	6
												2	−1	6	9	5
													−2	5	8	4
														8	11	3
															3	2

For explanations, see footnote to table 1.

Soldering problems and stress exerted on the electrode array may cause intermittent shorts and open electrodes that are not present during testing, or only at higher stimulation levels.

References

1 Game CJA, Thomson DR, Gibson WPR: Measurement of auditory brainstem responses evoked by electrical stimulation with a cochlear implant. Br J Audiol 1990;24:145–149.

2 Heller J, Brehm N, Sinopoli T, Shallop J: Characterization of surface-measured potentials from implanted cochlear prostheses. Proc IEEE EMBS Conf 1991;13: 1907–1908.

Dr. L.H.M. Mens, University Hospital Nijmegen St. Radboud, PO Box 9101, NL–6500 HB Nijmegen (The Netherlands)

Fraysse B, Deguine O (eds): Cochlear Implants: New Perspectives.
Adv Otorhinolaryngol. Basel, Karger, 1993, vol 48, pp 79–84

Comparative Reliability of Cochlear Implants

E.L. von Wallenberg[a], *J. Brinch*[b], *D.K. Money*[b], *R. West*[c], *K. Avunduk*[b]

[a]Cochlear AG, Basel, Switzerland; [b]Cochlear Pty. Ltd., Sydney, Australia; [c]Cochlear Corporation, Denver, Colo., USA

Cochlear implant reliability is important for patients and clinicians. We know that an internal device failure can be a traumatic experience for the patient, his family and the implant team. With some devices, there is more than 9 years of clinical experience available and comparisons of the reliability of the different cochlear implant designs are possible.

Reliability has been defined by the Electronics Industry Association in the USA as follows: 'Reliability is the probability of a device performing its purpose adequately for the period of time intended under the operating conditions.' The key elements of this definition focus on *performance, environment, time* and *probability. Performance,* in our case, means that the device meets its specification. The *environment* in which it has to perform is the human body. The desired *time* is the lifetime of the patient. Because, to date, the failure rate has been relatively small for those devices which have been implanted for a long time, it is hard to predict the *probability* for the implant to survive longer than our experience. The Cochlear company now has more than 9 years of experience with different models of cochlear implants. From the actual failure rate data at different device ages, the cumulative survival can be calculated which is a measure of the reliability. The cumulative survival shows the percentage of devices surviving to a certain age. Absolute numbers of failures would not be very meaningful because they do not take device age into account.

Before a new implant design is approved by our research and development team, many qualification tests are performed. Our experience in evaluating implant specifications has been recognized so that now some of these tests have been incorporated in the new European standard for active implantable medical devices (AIMD). Our environmental tests include: dry heat, cold temperature, free fall, thermal cycling, vibration, impact shock, electrode tests, failure-mode effect analysis and electromagnetic interference tests. Despite all of these tests which verify that the design meets the specification, device failures still may occur. In general, a device failure can be defined as 'the inability to perform its intended function'. We can differentiate between so-called *soft* and *hard* failures. *Soft* failures are characterized by a deviation from the specification without a total loss of function. In the case of the Nucleus cochlear implant these can be resolved through programming. For instance, electrode faults can be resolved by eliminating the electrode from the program in the speech processor. The *hard* failures involve the total loss of function and, therefore, require further surgery to remove and replace the implant. Fortunately, the smooth, tapered electrode array of the Nucleus device has proven relatively easy to replace and virtually all patients who have had device failures have been successfully revised.

There are different causes of failure which relate to the *design, manufacture* and *user. Design* refers to an inherent characteristic of the device. For example, using epoxy rather than hermetic packaging results in different failure rates. *Manufacturing*-induced failures are usually random defects introduced by component or process variations. A *user*-induced failure, for example, could be a severe blow to the implant site due to an accident.

For the following comparison of the reliability of the different cochlear implant designs, data on the hard failures will be discussed. The devices which were analyzed include two different designs of the Nucleus cochlear implant, as well as three 3M/House devices manufactured by the 3M company. 3M discontinued manufacturing cochlear implants in 1988. In August 1989 Cochlear bought the rights to their cochlear implants and took over the responsibility of servicing approximately 1,000 3M patients worldwide.

Materials and Methods

Data on two Nucleus implant designs were analyzed. The use of the Nucleus Standard implant began in 1982: it did not have a magnet. The Nucleus Mini System 22 was introduced in 1985 and had the same custom-integrated circuit [1]. The newer device is thinner and incorporates an internal magnet for the alignment of the external coil. Both devices are encapsulated in a hermetic titanium package and have a ceramic feed-through. The data on the number of implantations, as well as the failure rate data, is based on all reports received from the clinics as of 31.12.91.

The 3M/House device also underwent several design modifications [2]. The first design was an epoxy encapsulated receiver. The second and third 3M/House designs were both titanium encapsulated receivers. For the 3M devices, the reporting ended in December 1988 and, therefore, the data can only be shown up to that date.

If a device malfunction is suspected, surface potentials from the patient's head can be measured in order to verify the failure [3]. After explantation the device is returned to Cochlear for a detailed analysis of the failure mode.

The cumulative survival was calculated in the following way: All implant lifetimes are referenced to day zero when they were implanted [4]. Accumulated implant failures x_i are tabulated by the days to failure d_i with i being the index for each entry. The number of implants (number exposed) n_i which have survived until the lifetime (days to failure) d_i of a given number of implant failures x_i is established. Since the number of implants in the field is continuously growing the number of implants exposed decreases with increasing device age. The fraction of failed implants: $f_i = dx_i/n_i = (x_i - x_{i-1})/n_i$ is then calculated. The incremental survival is defined as $s_i = 1 - f_i$. Finally, the cumulative survival cs_i percentage is found from the equation: $cs_i = (s_i \times cs_{i-1}) \times 100$. For the graphic display of the cumulative survival, the incremental time period is selected. The cumulative survival percentage cs_i of the last failure (longest d_i) for a particular period is used to represent the entire period.

Results

As of December 1991, there had been 4,626 Nucleus devices implanted. The cumulative survival over device age for the two Nucleus devices and the 3M/House devices is plotted in figure 1 on a scale from 70 to 100% to allow direct comparison. A total of 448 Nucleus standard implants had been implanted with the longest implant duration being more than 9 years (111 months) and a cumulative survival at this device age of 92.8% (fig. 1a). The Nucleus Mini System 22 implant had been used for more than 6 years (76 months), a total of 4,178 devices had been implanted and the cumulative survival at this device life was 97.2% (fig. 1b).

Six hundred and twenty-four of the 3M/House epoxy receivers were implanted and the cumulative survival after 5.5 years was 73.4% (fig. 1c). The 3M/House second design was a titanium encapsulated receiver and 119 had been implanted. The cumulative survival was 87.1% after 2 years (fig. 1d). Subsequently, an improved third design was introduced

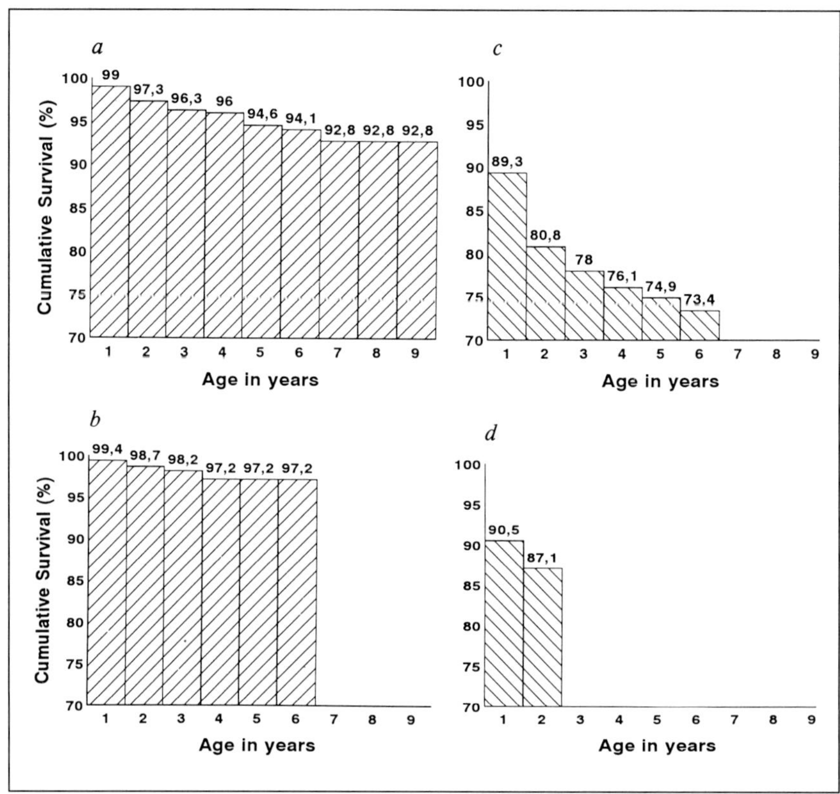

Fig. 1. Cumulative survival versus implant age in years: *a* Nucleus Standard implant. *b* Nucleus Mini System 22 implant. *c* 3M/House epoxy implant (1st design). *d* 3M/House titanium implant (2nd design). The data are as of 31.12.1991 for the Nucleus devices and as of 31.12.1988 for the 3M/House devices.

had a lower failure rate. A total of 276 of these devices had been implanted; however, there are only data for 1 year available, because 3M then stopped manufacturing cochlear implants.

In order to allow a better comparison of the reliability, the cumulative failures after 2 years have been tabulated for the different devices (table 1). The 2-year life span was selected because data for all implants, except for the third design of the 3M/House Titanium receiver, were available at this device age. The Nucleus device underwent a significant improvement from

Table 1. Comparison of cumulative failures (= 100% – cumulative survival) after 2 years (* 1 year) of implant age for five different implant designs

Implant type	Cumulative failures, %
Nucleus Mini System 22 Implant	1.33
Nucleus Standard Implant	2.73
3M/House Titanium Implant, 3rd design*	3.04
3M/House Titanium Implant, 2nd design	12.93
3M/House Epoxy Implant, 1st design	19.24

which 2.7% cumulative failure in the 1st design to 1.3% in the Mini System 22 implant. The nonhermetic 3M epoxy device had a cumulative failure rate which was more than ten times higher than that for the Mini implant.

Discussion

The data suggest that the majority of the failures in both Nucleus devices tend to occur earlier in the life of the devices, indicating that older implants may be less likely to fail. In the case of the 3M/House epoxy device, the cumulative survival is seen to be decreasing continuously with increasing device age. Furthermore, due to the nonhermetic encapsulation, these devices can be expected to fail prematurely. The 3M/House devices underwent a significant improvement with each re-design. The failure rate after 2 years (table 1) for the 3M/House Titanium second design was still approximately 10 times higher than for the Nucleus Mini System 22 Implant. The third design of the 3M/House Titanium device had a lower failure rate (3% after 1 year) than the earlier 3M devices.

Failure analysis of explanted devices and of manufacturing rejects enables the manufacturer to improve the product design and the manufacturing process over time. Cochlear continuously analyzes the different types of faults in the Nucleus device carefully and reviews the component or process involved in order to reduce the probability of future occurrences. This process is constantly improving the reliability of the Nucleus implant system.

Conclusion

The reliability of cochlear implants is increasing with design and process improvements. The earlier 3M epoxy cochlear implants failed prematurely. With the introduction of titanium packaging techniques, the reliability has grown considerably. The cumulative survival for the Nucleus Mini System 22 Implant is better than 97% after 6 years.

References

1 Clark GM, Blamey PJ, Brown AM, Gusby PA, Dowell RC, Franz BKH, Pyman BC, Shepherd RK, Tong YC, Webb RL, Hirshorn MS, Kuzma J, Mecklenburg DJ, Money DK, Patrick JFP, Seligman PM: The University of Melbourne – Nucleus Multi-Electrode Cochlear Implant; in Pfaltz CR (ed): Advances in ORL. Basel, Karger, 1987, vol 38, pp 63–84.

2 Danley MJ, Fretz RJ: Design and functioning of the single-electrode cochlear implant. Ann Otol Rhinol Laryngol 1982;91(suppl):21–26.

3 Heller J, Brehm N, Sinopoli T, Shallop JK: Characterization of surface-measured potentials from implanted cochlear prostheses. Proc IEEE EMBS Conf 1991;13: 1907–1908.

4 O'Connor PDT: Reliability Engineering. New York, Hemisphere, 1988.

Dr. E. von Wallenberg, Cochlear AG, Margarethenstrasse 47,
CH–4053 Basel (Switzerland)

Fraysse B, Deguine O (eds): Cochlear Implants: New Perspectives.
Adv Otorhinolaryngol. Basel, Karger, 1993, vol 48, pp 85–90

Comparison of Current Speech Coding Strategies

L.A. Whitford[a], *P.M. Seligman*[a], *P.J. Blamey*[b], *H.J. McDermott*[b], *J.F. Patrick*[a]

[a] Cochlear Pty Ltd., Sydney, and [b] Department of Otolaryngology, University of Melbourne, Australia

This paper reports on two studies carried out at the University of Melbourne jointly with Cochlear Pty Ltd. The studies demonstrated substantial speech perception improvements over the current Multipeak strategy in background noise.

'Characteristic Frequency' (Charf) Mapping

The first of these studies involves the use of standard Cochlear Pty Ltd. hardware and Multipeak strategy, but by altering the default frequency boundaries, attempts to map speech in a more natural position in the cochlea.

In the existing frequency to electrode allocation, generally all intracochlear electrodes producing auditory sensations are used, regardless of their position in the cochlea. While we assume that we are stimulating frequency regions between approximately 500 and 6,000 Hz in cases of a 25-mm insertion (when all active electrodes and stiffening rings are inside the scala tympani), this is not the case for shallower insertions.

For these shallower insertions, it is possible that there may be some benefit in concentrating the stimulation more apically. Blamey et al. [1], in an analysis of vowel confusion results, found that patients had a 'bias' towards responding with a vowel that had a higher second formant frequency than the stimulation, and this bias was related to the depth of insertion.

For this reason, it was decided to investigate a frequency mapping based on reported insertion depth of the electrode array, using characteristic frequency along the basilar membrane in a normal cochlea [2, 3].

It is clear that unless electrode insertion is sufficient to cover the frequency range down to the lowest frequency of the first formant, i.e. approximately 250 Hz, there are some compromises which must be made. For example, a patient with the most apical electrode at 21 mm from the round window would have a lowest frequency of stimulation of around 900 Hz. If we used a strict characteristic frequency allocation, this would effectively exclude all the speech information in the F1 frequency range. However, it has been shown that this information is important, with the F0F1F2 strategy providing substantial benefit over F0F2 [4].

At the other end of the array, the most basal electrode may lie at 20 kHz. However, the MSP (Mini Speech Processor, manufactured by Cochlear Pty Ltd.) only analyses speech to approximately 6 kHz. It is clear that some electrodes would be outside the normal range for speech. The question is therefore whether it is advantageous to use less than the maximum possible number of electrodes in an attempt to make speech sound more natural.

Mapping

To try to fulfill these conflicting requirements, we decided to investigate a frequency allocation which involved setting the frequency boundary for the electrode which has a characteristic frequency of approximately 3 kHz in the correct tonotopic position and allowing the DPS (diagnostic programming system) software to re-allocate all of the more apical electrodes to cover the whole of the F1 and F2 frequency ranges. This has the effect of shifting the F2 stimulation closer to the characteristic frequency region, while still maintaining a reasonable number of channels for F1 information.

The Multipeak speech processor (MSP) extracts the first and second formant and is also fitted with three fixed filters set at 2–2.8, 2.8–4 and 4–6 kHz. Electrodes in the F1 and F2 region are selected according to measured formant frequencies. The three fixed filters are allocated to three fixed basal electrodes. In ‘characteristic frequency’ mapping, the most basal electrode used is that which corresponds to the 5-kHz characteristic frequency region (based on the centre frequency of the highest filter).

Table 1. Patient results expressed as percent words correct for open-set sentences presented in background noise, for both Standard and Charf maps

Subject (depth)	Map	+5 dB S:N, %		+10 dB S:N, %		+15 dB S:N, %	
		mean	SD	mean	SD	mean	SD
S1	Std	40.3	7.3	73.8	6.9		
(20.5 mm)	Charf	50.8	8.4	88.5	2.6		
S2	Std	18.3	8.9	42.2	11.9		
(21 mm)	Charf	23.3	12.0	85.3	8.4		
S3	Std			40.5	10.7	71.3	7.2
(21 mm)	Charf			53.2	9.4	88.3	7.8
S4	Std	14.5	6.5	53.8	9.7		
(23.5 mm)	Charf	22.8	7.6	62.3	6.3		

Test Procedure and Results

Four postlinguistically deafened patients, all with insertion depths of at least 20 mm, participated in this study. These patients alternated between 'characteristic frequency' and standard mapping on a weekly or fortnightly basis (depending on how often they were able to come in for testing). At each of 8 sessions, they were tested with the program they had been using for the previous week or fortnight.

The patients were tested using CUNY [5] sentences presented in an open-set format at two signal-to-noise ratios between +5 and +15 dB (4-talker babble used as competing noise). The results are shown in table 1, together with the insertion depth for each patient. The mean score for each subject was higher for 'characteristic frequency' mapping than for standard mapping and this improvement was significant for each subject ($p < 0.05$, Wilcoxon matched-pairs).

The patients were also tested using monosyllabic word lists [6] recorded with both male and female speakers. While the mean word scores were always slightly higher for 'characteristic frequency' mapping than for standard mapping, this improvement was only significant for subject 2 (mean 66.0%, SD 9.9 for Charf mapping; mean 42.5%, SD 6.7 for standard mapping; $p < 0.001$, paired t test).

Modified Spectral Maxima Sound Processor (SMSP)

This work followed that reported earlier by McDermott et al. [7]. In their SMSP strategy, 16 bandpass filters are used, linearly spaced between 250 and 1,850 Hz and then logarithmically spaced up to 5,400 Hz. Each bandpass channel is allocated to its own electrode in the cochlea. Of the 16 channels, the 6 largest outputs are presented at a stimulation rate of 250 Hz. The filter energy is estimated by a full-wave rectifier followed by a 200-Hz low-pass filter.

In a modified implementation of the SMSP strategy (SPEAK), the amplitudes are extracted by an envelope tracking algorithm. This tracks the band-pass filter outputs without introducing any time-dependent processing. The six maxima are determined continuously rather than at the 4-ms intervals used previously. The amplitude mapping used is the same as is used in the MSP. The gains of the filter channels, as with the SMSP, are adjusted to approximately match the sensitivity of normal hearing.

A prototype bench-top processor implementing the SPEAK strategy in the MSP was produced and 3 patients were tested at the end of each of four test sessions. These patients also participated in the 'characteristic frequency' study (see above) and the earlier part of each session was devoted to that evaluation.

Test Procedure and Results

Prior to testing with the SPEAK strategy, the patients were given approximately 10 min practice with the strategy using auditory-alone speech tracking. Patient 4 was totally unfamiliar with the strategy; patients 1 and 2 had used the SMSP for approximately 3 months previously but had returned to using their normal speech processor (MSP) for at least 4 months prior to this study.

The patients were tested with six lists of open-set CUNY sentences at +5 dB signal-to-noise ratio (4-talker babble used as competing noise). The mean results of the testing in background noise are shown in table 2. Also shown are the results for these patients using 'characteristic frequency' mapping which were collected over the same period. The comparison is made with 'characteristic frequency' mapping, which for these patients was the best obtained with the MSP. The improvement in performance for this group of 3 subjects was significant ($p = 0.001$, paired t test).

The patients were also tested with a total of four lists of 50 monosyllabic words (200 words) in quiet. No significant differences were observed,

Table 2. Patient results for open-set sentences, presented in background noise at 5 dB SNR, comparing SPEAK and Charf maps

Subject	Strategy	+5 dB S:N, %	
		mean	SD
S1	SPEAK	82.0	4.6
	Charf	48.3	3.3
S2	SPEAK	57.0	11.2
	Charf	23.3	12.0
S4	SPEAK	21.7	5.6
	Charf	22.8	7.6
Total	SPEAK	50.0	25.9
	Charf	29.4	14.0

however it is possible that there would be an improvement on this test (which requires fine frequency discriminations) after patients had take-home experience with the device. Previous testing with the SMSP revealed a gradual improvement over time as patients gained experience with the strategy.

Conclusion

A group of 4 patients was tested with a strategy using standard hardware and modified mapping based on characteristic frequencies within the cochlea and showed significant improvement in open-set sentence recognition in relatively high levels of background noise. Three of these were further tested with a constant rate filter-bank strategy, and performance in noise showed an additional substantial improvement over that already obtained.

References

1 Blamey PJ, Whitford LA, Seligman PM, Clark G: Electrode identification and vowel recognition in cochlear implant patients. Abstr 14th Ann Meet Eur Neurosci Assoc, Cambridge, September 8–12. Eur J Neurosci 1991;(suppl 4):71.

2 Greenwood DD: Critical bandwidth and the frequency coordinates of the basilar membrane. J Acoust Soc Am 1961;33:1344–1356.
3 Greenwood DD: A cochlear frequency-position function for several species – 29 years later. J Acoust Soc Am 1990;87:2592–2605.
4 Dowell RC, Seligman PM, Blamey PJ, Clark GM: Evaluation of a two-formant speech-processing strategy for a multichannel cochlear prosthesis. Ann Otol Rhinol Laryngol 1987;96(suppl 128):132–133.
5 Boothroyd A, Hanin L, Hnath T: A sentence test of speech perception: Reliability, set equivalence, and short term learning. Internal Report no. RCI 10, Speech and Hearing Sciences Research Center, City University of New York, 1985.
6 Peterson G, Lehiste I: Revised CNC lists for auditory tests. J Speech Hear Disord 1962;27:62–70.
7 McDermott HJ, McKay CM, Vandali AE: A new portable sound processor for the University of Melbourne/Nucleus Ltd multi electrode cochlear implant. J Acoust Soc Am 1992;91:3367–3371.

Lesley Whitford, Cochlear Pty Ltd., 6th Floor, Royal Victoria Eye and Ear Hospital, 32, Gisborne Street, East Melbourne, Vic. 3002 (Australia)

Fraysse B, Deguine O (eds): Cochlear Implants: New Perspectives.
Adv Otorhinolaryngol. Basel, Karger, 1993, vol 48, pp 91–96

A Hybrid Coding Strategy for a Multichannel Cochlear Implant

W.K. Lai, N. Dillier, H. Bögli

Department of Otorhinolaryngology, University Hospital, Zurich, Switzerland

Results from two different speech coding strategies previously investigated by Bögli and Dillier [1] using the Melbourne-Nucleus cochlear implant have suggested that:

(i) A strategy (PES or pitch excited sampler) which presents the encoded information at a rate corresponding to the fundamental pitch frequency of the input speech signal is capable of producing good vowel identification, resonable consonant identification and not surprisingly, good voice pitch discrimination as well.

(ii) A strategy (CIS or continuous interleaved sampler) which presents the encoded information continuously to the implant at the maximum rate possible is capable of producing equally good vowel identification, improved consonant identification but virtually no voice pitch discrimination as this strategy does not specifically encode voice pitch information into the presented information.

The implication of the above was that the higher rate of stimulation associated with CIS is responsible for the improvements in consonant identification, while the specific coding of voice pitch information into the resultant stimuli is responsible for good voice pitch discrimination. To choose between the two strategies, however, would mean a compromise between consonant and voice pitch information transmission. Thus, in order to combine the positive characteristics of the two different strategies above, a number of hybrid variations of these two strategies were developed and investigated.

Method

The simplest hybrid tested involved using the absence or presence of voicing in the speech signal to select between CIS and PES stimulation, respectively. This was designated as the VS (voicing switched) hybrid.

If it is indeed more advantageous to present consonant information using CIS as suggested by the results from Bögli and Dillier, vowels could be presented with PES and consonants with CIS. To achieve this, a distinction has to be made between voiced consonants and vowels. Unvoiced consonants are simply indicated by the absence of voicing. Spectrograms of voiced consonants such as the voiced stops /b/, /d/ and /g/ indicated that the onset of these consonants are characterised by a second formant frequency that is relatively transitory compared to the more steady state vowel that follows in utterances such as /ba/, /da/ or /ga/. Thus, a second hybrid detected transitions in the F2 electrode trajectory to differentiate between voiced consonants and vowels. This hybrid, designated as the ETS (electrode trajectory switched) hybrid, thus attempts to present vowels using PES and consonants using CIS.

The two above hybrids alternate between PES or CIS stimulation according to some condition in the speech signal. A further hybrid variation would be to present CIS and PES stimulation simultaneously instead of alternating between them. Such hybrids (referred to here as integrated hybrids) could activate one or two of the lower frequency active electrodes using PES while the remaining higher frequency active electrodes would be activated using CIS. In the integrated hybrids presented here, unvoiced portions are presented using CIS only. Voiced portions are presented using the combined PES + CIS stimulation. This yields a voicing switched integrated hybrid, and two such hybrids, INT1V and INT2V, were investigated, the numeric label describing the number of lower frequency electrodes used for PES stimulation.

An obvious variation on the voicing switched integrated hybrid would be the electrode trajectory switched integrated hybrid, presenting voiced transient F2 portions in CIS. Two such hybrids, INT1E and INT2E, with one and two PES electrodes, respectively, were investigated.

A total of six hybrids were investigated in this study. Three of them, VS, INT1V and INT2V, are collectively referred to as the voicing sensitive hybrids, while the other three, ETS, INT1E and INT2E, are collectively referred to as the electrode trajectory sensitive hybrids.

Two tests were conducted to evaluate the relative performances of these hybrids:

(a) A Male-Female Speaker Identification Test, which involves identifying the speaker of a prerecorded sentence processed using the particular strategy as either male or female. Twenty prerecorded sentences were presented for identification by each participating cochlear implant user (implantee).

(b) A Rythme Test for Consonant Identification involving absolute identification of the middle consonant of common German bisyllabic words such as /leiber/, /leider/, /leiter/, /leiser/. A total of 100 words, involving 16 different middle consonants, were presented to each implantee for identification, each presentation involving a single-interval four-alternative forced-choice task. Pretest exposure of the implantee to each new strategy simply involved presenting conversational speech through the selected strategy for ten minues or so, followed by a simple number identification test using randomised prerecorded numbers (spoken in German) between 30 and 99.

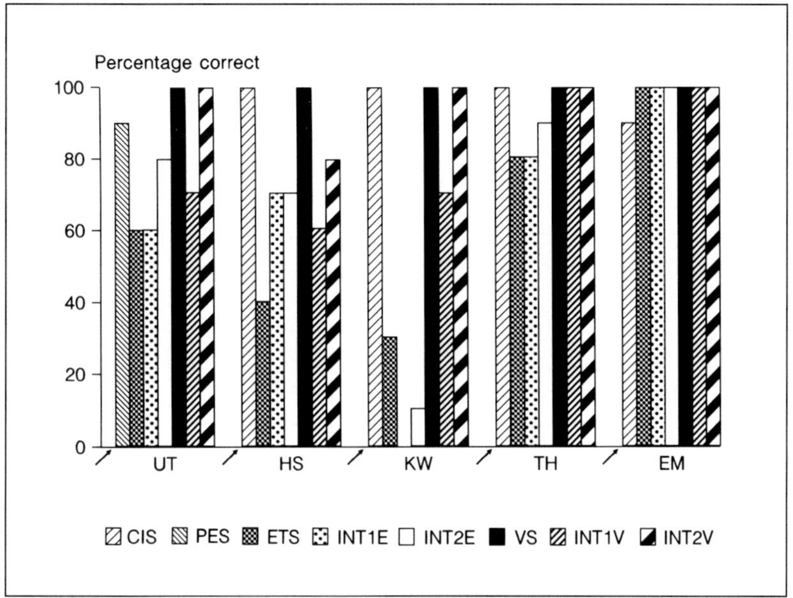

Fig. 1. Chance level corrected scores for the Male-Female Speaker Identification Test for all five implantees. Note that CIS scores (indicated by the arrows) were all zero.

In order to provide a more comprehensive comparison of these hybrids, results from PES and CIS previously collected for the same two tests with the same implantees are also presented here.

A total of five implantees took part in evaluating each of the various strategies. Data for all five implantees are presented for the first test, while only data for four implantees are presented with the second test as the fifth implantee had not completed all strategies at the time of this writing.

All data was collected in the form of confusion matrices before being subjected to analysis.

Results

Figure 1 summarizes the chance level corrected identification scores from the Male-Female Speaker Identification Test. The results for CIS, indicated by arrows, were all zero. All implantees obtained good speaker identification socres with all hybrids except KW with the ETS hybrid.

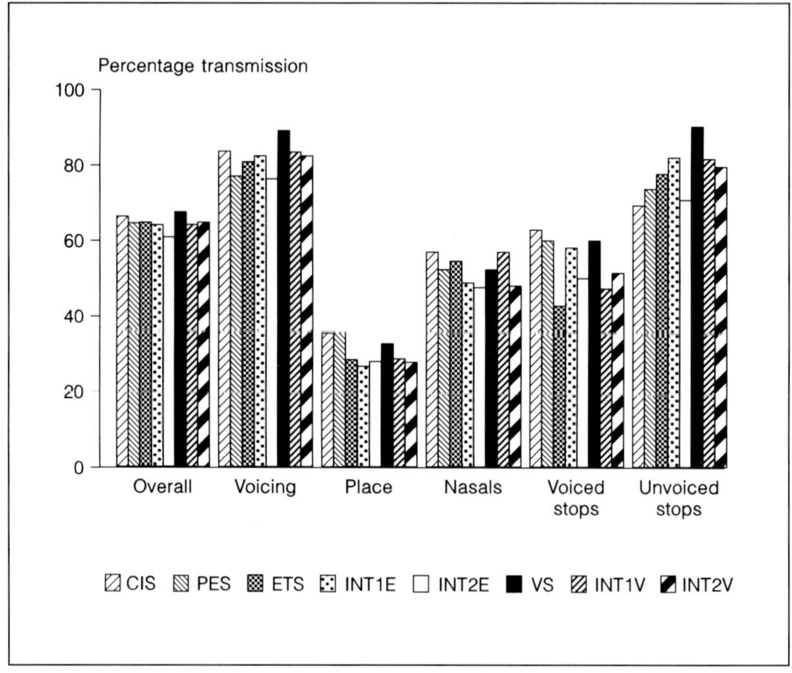

Fig. 2. Information transmission analysis results for various consonant features including the overall amount of information transmitted.

The result from the Rhyme Test were subjected to information transmission analysis (after Miller and Nicely [2]) for transmission of a number of different consonant features such as voicing, place of articulation, nasality, voiced stops and unvoiced stops. These results, summarised in figure 2, showed little difference between all eight strategies compared in the overall amount of information transmitted. Improved transmission was obtained for the voicing feature with the voicing sensitive hybrids, VS, INT1V and INT2V. Little difference was observed for the transmission of the place of articulation feature. The voicing sensitive hybrids indicated better transmission of the unvoiced stops /p/, /t/ and /k/ compared to PES and CIS. However, there was no difference between all strategies in transmission of the nasals /m/, /n/ and /9/, and poorer transmission of the voiced stops /b/, /d/ and /g/ with all hybrids compared to PES and CIS.

Discussion

The above results should be regarded only as preliminary, given the relatively small number of participating implantees. However, the Male-Female Speaker Identification Test results suggest that the presence of specific voice pitch coding in the form of PES stimulation is possibly sufficient to achieve a reasonable degree of voice pitch transmission. The results also indicate that, in general, two PES electrodes were able to transmit voice pitch information better than only one PES electrode although this difference was not very great.

Although the overall amount of information did not appear to differ much across all eight strategies, a closer look at the transmission of the various features showed a more interesting picture. The improved voicing feature transmission with a number of the hybrids is possibly due to a greater distinction between voiced and unvoiced portions due to switching between PES/PES + CIS and CIS only stimulation. On the other hand, the transmission of the place of articulation feature is not so easy to interpret. Closer examination showed that unvoiced consonants were better identifed with the hybrids, particularly the voicing sensitive hybrids. With the voicing sensitive hybrids, all these unvoiced stop consonants would have been presented using CIS, suggesting that the CIS mode of stimulation is useful for presenting such consonant information. With the Electrode Trajectory Sensitive Hybrids, the CIS portions would last a little longer due to the transient F2 trajectory expected at the vowel onset immediately following the unvoiced stop consonant. It would thus seem that this little extra CIS stimulation has an influence on the perception of these consonants. With the voiced stops, however, all hybrids generally fared poorer than either PES or CIS. The electrode trajectory sensitive hybrids were designed particularly with the intention of presenting the dynamic formant transitions of these voiced consonants, and it appears that this has not been successful, although the reason remains obscure. Also, the nasals showed little difference in identification between all strategies compared. It is not clear from this data exactly why the hybrids did not produce improved identification of these voiced consonants. Perhaps the switching between various stimulation modes such as CIS only, PES only and PES + CIS produces some sensations which interfere with the perception of the information characteristic to these voiced consonants. Psychophysical tests will have to be conducted to determine the nature of the sensations associated with these hybrids before a clear explanation can be offered for this observation.

Conclusions

The results from the Male-Female Speaker Identification test indicate that it is possible to present voice pitch information in essentially CIS-like strategies such as the integrated hybrids by using PES stimulation. The long-term physiological effects of chronic stimulation with CIS-like strategies is still unknown, and these hybrid strategies offer a possibility of avoiding continuous high rate stimulation. A secondary effect of this is that some savings in power consumption can also be achieved. The hybrid strategies were also able to marginally improve transmission of the voicing and frication features in consonants, probably due to the greater distinction between voiced and unvoiced portions of speech as a result of switching between PES and CIS. The effectiveness of CIS in transmitting consonant information in the hybrids is also indicated by the improved unvoiced stop consonant identification. However, further tests will have to be carried out to systematically determine the nature of the perceptual sensations related to the hybrid stimuli in order to achieve a better understanding of how the hybrid designs can be used to improve transmission of speech information.

References

1 Bögli H, Dillier N: Digital speech processor for the Nucleus 22-channel cochlear implant. Proc 13th Ann Int Conf IEEE/EMBS 1991, vol 13, pp 1901–1902.
2 Miller GA, Nicely P: An analysis of perceptual confusions among some English consonants. J Acoust Soc Am 1955;27:338–352.

Dr. W.K. Lai, Department of Otorhinolaryngology, University Hospital, CH–8091 Zurich (Switzerland)

Electrophysiology

Fraysse B, Deguine O (eds): Cochlear Implants: New Perspectives.
Adv Otorhinolaryngol. Basel, Karger, 1993, vol 48, pp 97–102

Significance of the Promontory Test: Histological and Electrical Results

M.J. Estève-Fraysse, G. Corvera, O. Deguine, A. Sans, M. Vincent, D. Laur, F. Sonilhac

CHU Purpan, Toulouse, France

The promontory test is a psychoacoustic test which tends to evaluate the capacity of the cochlear system to respond to electrical stimulation. So far, histological studies have demonstrated the persistence of numerous ganglion cells in deaf patients as well as in patients after cochlear implantation and labyrinthectomy. In parallel, the promontory test gives similar responses in profoundly deaf patients of varied etiology, and in labyrinthectomy patients.

In our work, we have tried to ascertain the role of cochlear nerve fibers during peripheral electrical stimulation.

Material and Methods

Thirty patients presenting with acoustic neuroma had a promontory test before surgery. The results were correlated with audiometric and electrophysiological data. Then, in 7 of these patients, in order to compare electrical and histological data, we studied the promontory test and the histology of the cochlear nerve which was removed during surgery using the translabyrinthine approach (when invasion of the nerve by the tumor was suspected). Finally, 5 of these patients were tested from 2 weeks to 3 months postoperatively.

Protocol

The promontory test was carried out by placing a transtympanic needle with sinusoidal stimulation in which we vary the intensity, measured in microamperes and millivolts. We look for (1) the minimum threshold perceived, and (2) the maximum acceptable level at these frequencies from 125, 250, 500, 1,000, 2,000 and 4,000 Hz.

Table 1. Dynamic mean values: Endocochlear/retrocochlear deafness

Frequencies, Hz	Preimplantation (19 cases)	Acoustic neurome (30 cases)
125	7.12 ± 1.63	4.28 ± 2.61
250	6.3 ± 4.8	4.66 ± 3.2
500	4.3 ± 4.7	5.56 ± 3.3
1,000	1.91 ± 5.53	4.51 ± 2.5
2,000	1.81 ± 4.78	4.48 ± 3.3
4,000	2.37 ± 3.21	3.38 ± 2.57

We look also for the dynamic range, which is expressed in decibels by the formula:

$$20 \log \frac{\text{maximum acceptable level}}{\text{minimum threshold}},$$

to minimize individual variations. Finally, we perform a sensory discrimination test to determine the minimum time between two stimulations that a patient can perceive.

Results

We present the dynamic mean values by frequency.

It appears firstly that the values are homogenous over all frequencies (table 1), and secondly that no significant statistical correlation is found between dynamic values or threshold of the promontory test versus either the average audiometric hearing loss, the i.v. delay in ABR, or the N1 wave of electrocochleography.

If we compare these results with those of 19 profoundly deaf patients during assessment of implantation we see that a different profile of dynamic range exists in endocochlear versus retrocochlear deafness.

Endocochlear deafness presents the best results at low frequencies: 1.25, 2.50, and 500 Hz (table 1). These frequencies correspond to segment IV of Koenig's scale and Schuknecht has shown that the density of the ganglion cells is highest here and that this region is less sensitive to age and different pathologies (fig. 1).

Let's look at the correlation of the promontory test and the histology of the cochlear nerve.

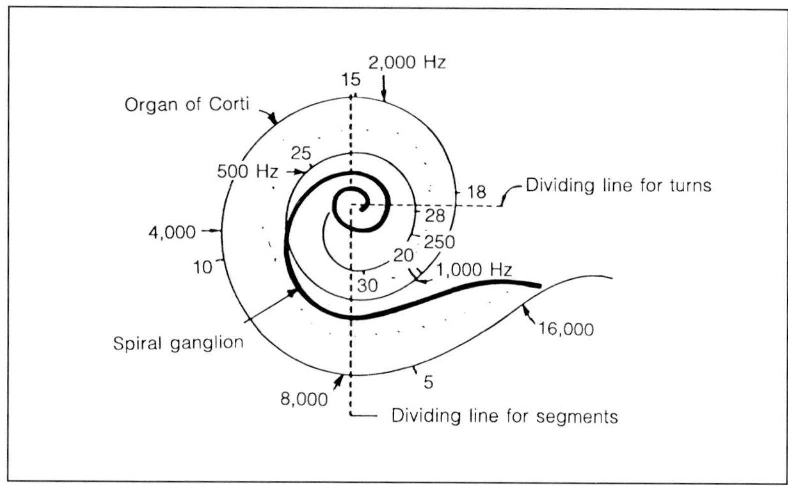

Fig. 1.

Segment	Length of ganglion mm	Ganglion of Corti, mm		Approximate frequency range, Hz	Percent of total ganglion cells
		region	length		
I	4.2	0–6	6	20,000–8,000	15
II	4.3	6–15	9	8,000–2,000	37
III	1.8	15–22	7	2,000–900	20
IV	1.7	22–32	10	900–0	28
Total	12	32	32	20,000–0	100

After Otte and Schuknecht, Laryngology, August 1978.

The histological studies were done in the laboratory of Prof. Sans in Montpellier.

They were done in semifine slices, with an ultramicrotome of 1 μm. The nerve was placed in Araldite, colored toluidine blue with photo enlargement and manual count. In several slices, an undifferentiated mass, probably representing tumor invasion, can be observed. The count was done on the most spherical slices with the least tumor invasion. Only fibers with an axoplasm surrounded by a myelin sheath were counted, some were the size of the fibers. To make the results uniform and because the size of

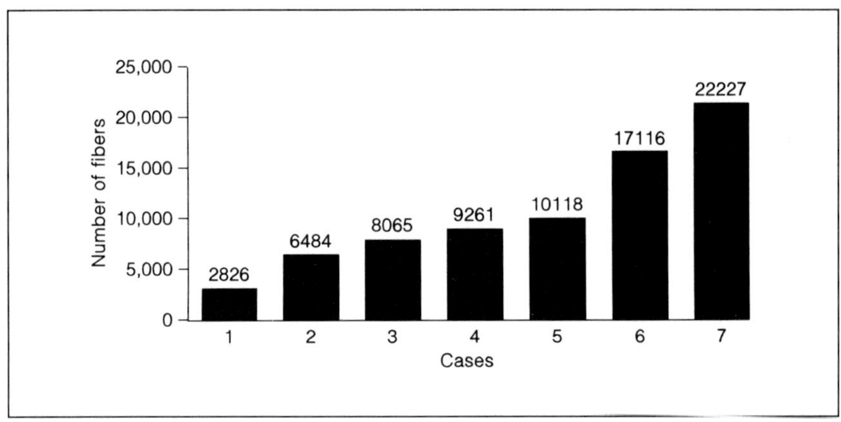

Fig. 2. Number of fibers of cochlear nerve/mm^2.

samples varied by a few millimeters, all of our results will be represented by number of fibers per 1 mm^2.

In figure 2 one can see that the number of fibers for our 7 patients varies between 2,800 and 22,000.

Otte and Schuknecht showed that the number of fibers is 36,000 at birth, and decreases by 2,000 every 10 years.

For each patient we calculated the number of fibers which is normal in relation to age (table 2) and then the percentage of counted fibers in relation to the normal number of fibers by age. The result varies from 11 to 84%.

In table 3, we compare the percent of fibers present and the dynamic range. It can be seen that when the percentage of fibers was higher than 75%, the mean dynamic range was highest at 6 dB, however, that is not statistically significant perhaps due to the smaller number of patients. Below this point, the results are varied. We then reported the values of mean dynamic for low, middle and high frequencies, and again these are shown according to the number of fibers (table 4). We correlated these mean dynamics with the number of fibers and we found a significant correlation at low and high frequencies but not at middle frequencies. These correlation seem to suggest that the dynamic range is proportional to the number of fibers present.

Table 2. Number and percent of fibers in relation to age

Case No.	Age, years	Number of fibers/age	Percent of fibers/age
1	54	25,000	11
2	38	28,000	23
3	68	22,000	36
4	45	27,000	37
5	58	24,000	38
6	72	22,000	77
7	49	26,000	85

Table 3. Percent of fibers/mean dynamic

Case No.	% of fibers	Mean dynamic/frequency, dB
1	11	3.9
2	23	5.86
3	36	3.92
4	37	3.07
5	38	4.78
6	77	6.78
7	85	6.19

Table 4. Dynamics by frequency

Case No.	Dynamics		
	125–250 Hz*	500–1,000 Hz	2,000–4,000**
1	0	5.53	1.34
2	5.34	9.13	3.11
3	5.4	2.55	3.8
4	2.88	4.42	1.91
5	3.73	5.57	5.03
6	6.16	8.33	5.84
7	8.13	4.42	6.02

* p = 0.01; ** p = 0.02.

Finally, it is important to note, in 5 of these patients where the promontory test was done 2 weeks to 3 months postoperatively, that none of them responded. Only pain responses were found.

Conclusion

Our results show: (1) A different profile of promontory test in retrocochlear deafness with homogeneous dynamic values at all frequencies. (2) They suggest that the promontory test is not an all or nothing test, but there is a relationship exists between the number of fibers and the dynamic range at low and high frequencies.

Finally, this test does not correlate with the audiometric and electrophysiological results.

Dr. M.J. Estève-Fraysse, CHU Purpan, Place du Docteur-Baylac,
F–31059 Toulouse Cedex (France)

Fraysse B, Deguine O (eds): Cochlear Implants: New Perspectives.
Adv Otorhinolaryngol. Basel, Karger, 1993, vol 48, pp 103–107

Preoperative Electrical Nerve Stimulation as One of the Criteria for Selection

J.E. Van Dijk, A.F. van Olphen, G.F. Smoorenburg

Department of Otorhinolaryngology, University Hospital Utrecht, The Netherlands

In several institutes electrical nerve stimulation is used as a preoperative diagnostic. The most important question is whether or not the auditory nerve and higher cortical functions are still intact. Especially the amount of degeneration of the acoustic nerve is the subject of investigation. In addition, the outcomes of electrical nerve stimulation are used to predict whether or not the patient will benefit from the implant. Although electrical stimulation of the auditory nerve has been performed in many institutes for several years, the significance of this test still seems to be limited.

Methods

In 1987 we presented our first results of preoperative electrostimulation [1]. The electrode was positioned at the promontory (P), in the round window niche (R), or at a position along the line P-R at about a quarter of the distance P-R from the round window (position Q). At these positions thresholds and loudness discomfort levels (LDLs) were measured between 63 Hz and 2 kHz (with intervals of half an octave). At 2/3 of the dynamic range above threshold, patients were asked to describe the sound they experienced. The dynamic range appeared to increase from P to Q and from Q to R. Therefore, all later tests were performed with the electrode placed at position Q. Only if the results were not satisfactory was the tympanic membrane opened under local anesthesia and a ball-electrode was placed at position R.

We also measured the temporal resolution by presenting two tone bursts, separated by a silent interval of 500 ms. The first tone burst was 300 ms in duration, the second 300 + T ms. The task was to discriminate (20 times for every T value) between the duration of the two bursts. T values between 60 and 200 ms were used. The score is the number of

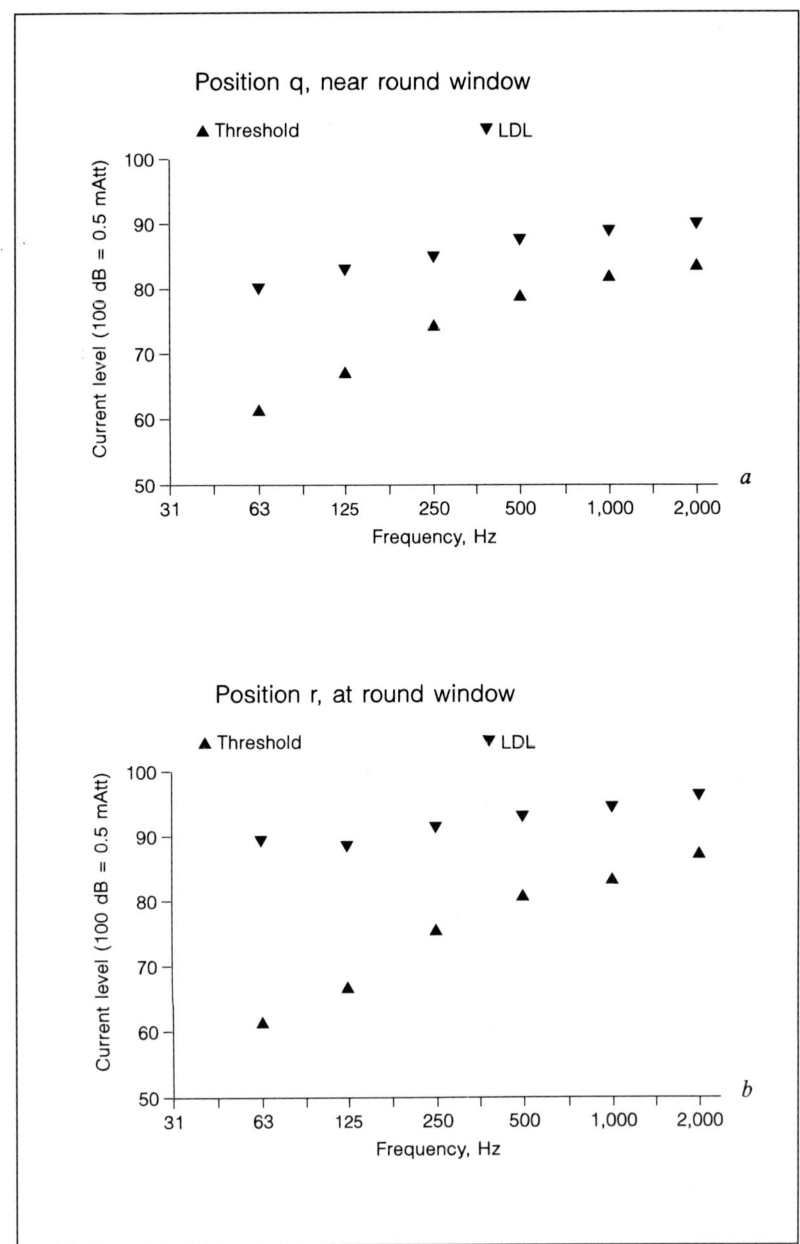

Fig. 1. Average preoperative threshold and LDL values measured *(a)* near the round window (n = 49) and *(b)* at the round window (n = 12).

correct responses; a score of 10 corresponds to chance. We derived a new parameter, the sound identification score (SI score), from the sound description the patients reported while measuring the dynamic range. If the discrimination between the different frequencies was very poor SI = 1, if the patient could discriminate between all frequencies SI = 5.

Results

Dynamic Range

In figure 1 the thresholds and LDLs are presented for the positions Q (n = 49 ears) and R (n = 12). Some increase of dynamic range, although not significant, was found from Q to R. Ship and Nedzelski [2] described the same effect (also not significant) between promontory and round window electrode positions.

At position Q, at low frequencies (63 and 125 Hz) the dynamic range diminished with increasing threshold values, correlation coefficient r = −0.73. There is only a poor correlation (r = 0.29) between the dynamic range and the LDL values. This means that the main component in the dynamic range is the threshold. At high frequencies (1 kHz) all ears appear to have relatively high thresholds and low dynamic ranges.

Dynamic Range and Other Preoperative Measures

In the upper part of figure 2, it can be seen that there is no relation between the dynamic range and temporal resolution (r = 0.06).

For the SI score in the lower part of figure 2, we did find some relation to dynamic range. The SI score was always low (0–3) for dynamic ranges below 12 dB (at 125 Hz); at higher dynamic ranges, SI scores from 1 to 5 were found.

Preoperative Measures versus Postoperative Results

Patients who received a 3M single-channel device were asked to perform a simple test in which they had to recognize numbers from one to ten. In table 1, the results of this test are compared to the preoperative dynamic range at 125 Hz (position Q), temporal resolution score at T = 60 ms and the SI score. Patients with a Nucleus 22 channel system were presented with a more difficult task; they had to respond to an open set of CVC words. In table 2 the phoneme score in % is compared to the preoperative measures.

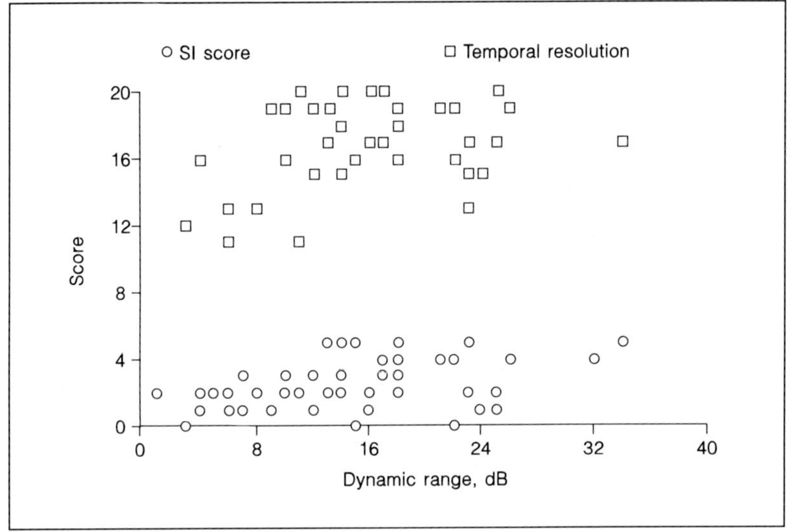

Fig. 2. Temporal resolution score (10–20; 10 is chance) at 60 ms and sound identification score (SI = 1–5) as a function of the dynamic range. SI score zero denotes no measurement.

Table 1. Patients with a 3M single channel device

	Patient No.					
	1	2	3	4	5	6
Dynamic range, dB	21	14	10	14	25	27
Temporal resolution, %	95	90	95	100	100	100
SI score (1–5)	3	–	3	5	1	–
Number recognition, %	83	22	11	61	0	0

Conclusions

We found little correlation among the preoperative measures: dynamic range, temporal resolution and sound identification score.

Patients with good preoperative results may have good, but also poor postoperative results.

Table 2. Patients with a Nucleus 22 channel device

	Patient No.			
	7	8	9	10
Dynamic range, dB	13	18	23	25
Temporal resolution, %	95	95	75	85
SI score (1–5)	2	4	5	2
Phoneme recognition, %	50	34	25	10

It is striking that the phoneme score in the Nucleus patients increases with a decreasing preoperative dynamic range.

However, since no patients with poor preoperative electrostimulation results were implanted, one should be cautions in drawing conclusions from the present data.

References

1 Smoorenburg GF, van Olphen AF: Pre-operative electrostimulation of the auditory nerve and post-operative results with the House/3M cochlear implant. Cochlear Implant Symp, 1987, Düren, p 227.

2 Ship DB, Nedzelski JM: Round window versus promontory stimulation: Assessment for cochlear implant candidacy. Ann Otol Rhinol Laryngol 1991;100:889–892.

J.E. Van Dijk, Department of Otorhinolaryngology, University Hospital, F.02.504, P.O. Box 85500, NL–3508 GA Utrecht (The Netherlands)

Fraysse B, Deguine O (eds): Cochlear Implants: New Perspectives.
Adv Otorhinolaryngol. Basel, Karger, 1993, vol 48, pp 108–113

Ear Canal Electrodes versus Promontory Electrodes in Preoperative Electrical Stimulation for Cochlear Implant Selection

T.H. Spies, A.F.M. Snik, L.H.M. Mens, P. van den Broek

University Hospital Nijmegen St. Radboud, Nijmegen, The Netherlands

In most cochlear implant centres a preoperative electrostimulation of the ear is performed to verify whether the candidate experiences hearing sensations while stimulated electrically. In some studies correlations have been reported between results on the preoperative electrostimulation and postoperative performance scores [1–3] but correlations are found to be poor in other studies [4]. Unfortunately, these studies are not easy to compare because of differences in the preoperative stimulation methods (e.g. the type of stimulus used, the location of the stimulating electrodes, including or excluding prelingually deafened subjects, the definition of a 'positive' electrostimulation). It is not even clear whether the absence of hearing sensations on preoperative electrostimulation necessarily implies that the patient will not benefit from the implant.

The present study deals with the difference between preoperative promontory stimulation and stimulation in the ear canal with respect to the number of ears in which hearing sensations are evoked and on the threshold and dynamic range values.

Electrostimulation on the promontory is more commonly used because the electrode position is relatively close to the cochlea. However, several authors have indicated the usefulness of the ear canal is a location for electrode placement [5–7]. An ear canal electrode typically consists of a metal wire hanging in saline solution, which fills the ear canal. Claimed advantages are the ease of placement and the relative insensitivity of the test results to small variations in the location of the electrode [5]. On the other hand, high current levels are needed because of the relatively large distance of an ear canal electrode to the auditory nerve. This easily gives rise to unwanted somatosensory sensations.

Methods

Patients

Forty-three postlingually deafened CI candidates (22 men and 21 women) were submitted to preoperative electrostimulation (ECS and/or PS). Their ages varied from 13 to 70 with a mean of 45.8 years. Meningitis was the most common cause of deafness (14), followed by hereditary causes (11) and head trauma (6). Chronic otitis, otosclerosis and Ménière's disease contributed in 2 cases each and 6 times no cause for the deafness could be found.

Materials

The output of the current source was independent from output impedance up to 30 V output voltage. The maximum output current was set at 1.4 mA (0 dB reference level). The electrical stimuli were sinewave bursts of 500-ms duration.

Procedure

The needle-electrode, used for PS, had a ball-shaped tip with a diameter of 0.6 mm. Following paracentesis, the tip was placed on the promontory in the vicinity of the round window niche. The ear canal electrode used was a plastic V-shaped spring (commercially available as 'Eartrode' for electrocochleography). After removal of excessive cerumen, checking the intactness of the ear drum and moisturizing the ear canal with a 0.9% saline solution, the electrode was placed using a small amount of electrode paste. The tip of the electrode was positioned close to the tympanic membrane without touching it. A reference electrode was positioned on the skin of the mastoid process. In a pilot study, several locations on the head for the reference electrode were tried and compared. No differences in threshold or produced sensations were found, except for a postition inside the contralateral ear canal, which resulted in bilateral hearing sensations. Patients were seated in a comfortable chair.

Threshold (T) and discomfort (D) levels were determined for each frequency using standard audiometrical procedures. The T level was defined as the minimum current that gave a hearing sensation with certainty. The sensation was considered to be a hearing sensation if the patient claimed that the stimulus was heard and adequately described a tonal quality as opposed to a (additional) tactile quality. The D level was defined as the current level at which the sensation was beginning to become very unpleasant.

Results

The reported sensations were classified as 'hearing' or, if no hearing was reported, as 'feeling only'. Hearing was often described as humming, buzzing or ringing. No significant differences in quality of the perceived

Table 1. Sensations evoked by promontory stimulation and ear canal stimulation in 43 postlingually deafened CI candidates

	Hearing	Feeling	Total
PS	38	6	44
ECS	42	9	51
Total	80	15	95

Values are the number of ears.

sounds evoked by PS or ECS were reported. Table 1 shows that PS did not produce hearing sensations in 6 ears (14%) and ECS in 9 ears (18%).

Results from ECS and PS in the same ears (n = 19) were compared. In all ears in which ECS produced a hearing sensation (in 16 of the 19 ears), PS did too. In 2 ears, both ECS and PS failed to produce hearing sensations. However, in 1 ear ECS did not lead to hearing, whereas PS did.

Stimuli of high frequency appeared less effective in producing hearing sensations than low-frequency stimuli, i.e., T levels grew steeper with frequency than D levels (fig. 1); furthermore, in 6 ears (12%) no D level for ECS was found at the 0-dB limit of the current source. In figure 2 the percentage of ears in which a hearing sensation could be evoked at a particular stimulus frequency is presented.

The mean T levels and electrical dynamic ranges (EDR) obtained in ECS and PS at 62 and 125 Hz are given in table 2. Because of the small number of ears with hearing sensations at high stimulus frequencies, only data from 62 and 125 Hz are given. The T levels and EDR values are significantly higher for PS than for ECS (Student's t test, $p < 0.05$).

Reinsertion of the ear canal electrode was performed in 6 ears. The mean T level at the lower frequencies (20 measurements) was not significantly better after reinsertion (0.45 dB, SD 2.1 dB).

Discussion

ECS as well as PS proved to evoke sensations that were claimed to be of auditory origin in most deaf cochlear candidates. ECS evoked hearing sensations in 82% of the ears and PS in 86% (table 1). This is in good

1
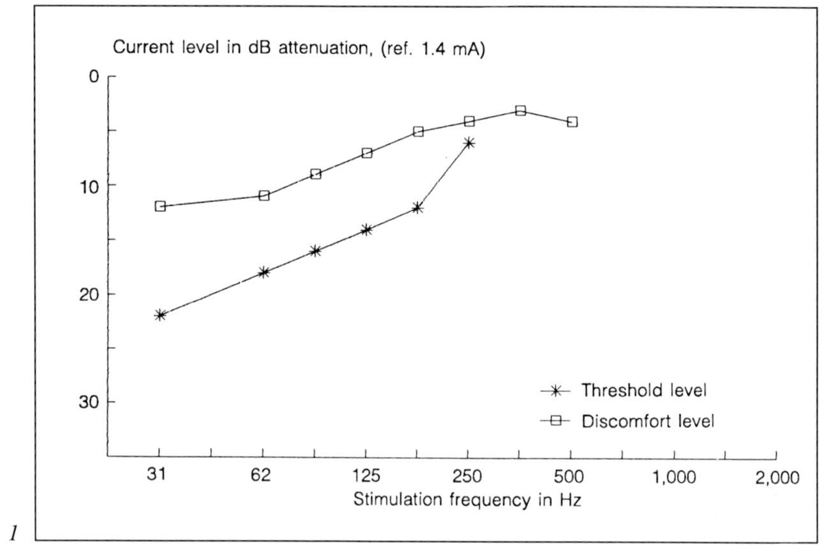

2
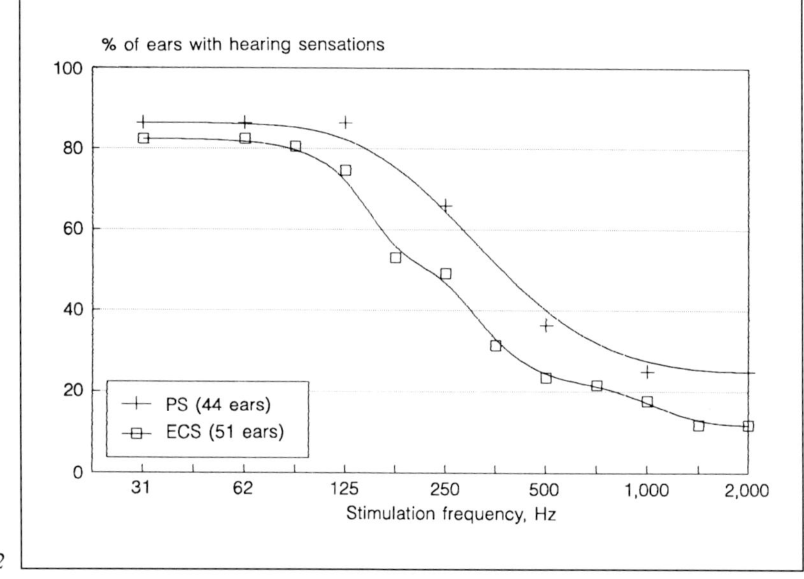

Fig. 1. A typical example of T and D levels in a postlingually deafened subject stimulated by an ear canal electrode. Separate observations are connected with lines. The area between the lines for T and D level represents the EDR.

Fig. 2. The relation between the stimulus frequency and the percentage of the stimulated ears in which hearing sensations were evoked.

Table 2. Mean threshold and electrical dynamic range at 62 and 125 Hz in promontory stimulation and in ear canal stimulation

	PS (n = 44 ears)		ECS (n = 51 ears)	
	mean	SD	mean	SD
Threshold, 62 Hz	45.8	6.4	17.7	3.9
Threshold, 125 Hz	39.7	6.5	12.7	4.4
Electric dynamic range, 62 Hz	15.6	5.8	10.0	3.8
Electric dynamic range, 125 Hz	12.6	5.1	6.5	3.1

Threshold in dB attenuation; electrical dynamic range in dB.

agreement with results from other goups that also use stimulus bursts of continuous waves [5, 7, 8]. The present results suggest that ECS and PS produce hearing sensations about equally often. From the 19 ears we stimulated with both methods, in only one ear PS resulted in hearing whereas ECS did not.

The mean T level at 62 Hz proved to be lowest in PS, and 28.1 dB higher in ECS. This difference is statistically significant and indicates that the proportion of the current actually reaching the auditory nerve is much smaller in ECS than in PS. The mean T level in ECS corresponds very well with data derived from Burian and Klasek [1]. The mean EDR was significantly poorer in ECS than in PS.

The application of the electrode in ECS appeared to be easier, required less preparation and organisation and was therefore less time consuming than the placement of a needle electrode for PS. Most patients found ECS less frightening when announced and were less nervous when the electrode was placed. Afterwards, however, the placement of a needle electrode was considered tolerable as well. Because of the noninvasiveness, the ease of application and the adequate reproducibility, ECS can also be used for repetitive measurements and allows interruption of the investigation. The traditional ECS with the salt solution in the ear canal requires the ear canal to be nearly vertical to precent the salt solution leaking out. This orientation of the head has a detrimental effect on lipreading. We therefore prefer the procedure with the clip electrode, in which the subject is allowed to sit up.

Conclusion

ECS proved an easily applicable noninvasive method with which hearing sensations could be evoked in most ears of a population of postlingually deafened CI candidates. Although a positive ECS was always accompanied by a positive PS, a negative ECS did not exclude hearing sensations from occurring in PS.

References

1 Burian K, Klasek O: Prognostische Hinweise im Rahmen der Selektion von Cochlearimplantatpatienten. Laryngol Rhinol Otol 1989;68:221–224.

2 Waltzmann SB, Cohen NL, Shapiro WH, Hoffman RA: The prognostic value of round window electrical stimulation in cochlear implant patients. Otolaryngol Head Neck Surg 1990;103:102–106.

3 Kileny PR, Kemink JL, Zimmerman-Phillips S, Schmaltz SP: Effects of preoperative electrical stimulability and historical factors on performance with multichannel cochlear implant. Ann Otol Rhinol Laryngol 1991;100:563–568.

4 Gantz BJ, Tyler RS, Knutson JF, Woodworth G, Abbas P, McCabe BF, Hinrichs J, Tye-Murray N, Lansing C, Kuk F, Brown C: Evaluation of five different cochlear implant designs: Audiologic assessment and predictors of performance. Laryngoscope 1988;98:1100–1106.

5 Dillier NT, Spillmann B: Ergebnisse der elektrischen Stimulation beim Normalhörenden, Schwerhörigen und Gehörlosen. Aktuelle Probleme der Otorhinolaryngologie. Bern, Huber, 1978, vol 1.

6 Schorn K, Seifert J, Stecker M, Zollner M: Voruntersuchungen gehörloser Patienten zur Cochlea-Implantation. Laryngol Rhinol Otol 1986;65:114–117.

7 Burian K, Hochmair-Desoyer IJ, Klasek O: Comparison of stimulation via transtympanic promontory electrodes, implanted electrodes and saltelectrodes in the earcanal. Int Cochlear Implant Symp, Düren, 1987, pp 157–160.

8 House WF, Brackmann DE: Electrical promontory testing in differential diagnosis of sensori-neural hearing impairment. Laryngoscope 1974;84:2163–2171.

Dr. L.H.M. Mens, University Hospital Nijmegen St. Radboud, PO Box 9101, NL–6500 HB Nijmegen (The Netherlands)

Fraysse B, Deguine O (eds): Cochlear Implants: New Perspectives.
Adv Otorhinolaryngol. Basel, Karger, 1993, vol 48, pp 114–119

Is the Round-Window Electrical Test Possible in Children?

E. Truy, A. Morgon, L. Collet, J.M. Chanal, A.M. Jonas, J. Girard, C. Berger-Vachon

Service d'Oto-Rhino-Laryngologie, de Chirurgie Cervico-Faciale et de Phoniatrie, Hôpital Edouard-Herriot, Lyon, France

Cochlear implantation in young children is currently the only hope in the case of total deafness. Pre-implantation testing is absolutely necessary for a good indication and to help establish a prognosis for prosthetic rehabilitation. The problems induced by pre-implantation electrical testing in children are not yet all solved.

(1) The electrical tests (such as the promontory or the round-window stimulation) can't be done routinely in children without general anesthesia because they need a surgical transmeatal approach.

(2) The subjective electrical tests can't be done easily in very young children because it is not always easy to get them to cooperate.

(3) The electrically evoked auditory brainstem responses (E-EABRs) are difficult to obtain because of the presence of the stimulus artefact.

We tried to better predict the quality of prosthetic rehabilitation in children by using some electrical tests. The goal is to test the ability of the remaining nervous fibers to be excited. These tests are done after the temporary implantation of an electrode through the round window, and are integrated with all classical tests such as otological, audiological, morphological by tomodensitometry, and psychological. In this way, we tried to obtain predicting factors.

Methods

Subjects

The study involved 6 patients aged from 2 to 14 years, they all were pre- or peri-linguistically deaf children. There were 4 girls and 2 boys with total bilateral deafness without useful benefit of an acoustical hearing aid. The parents' consent was always obtained.

Electrode Implantation

The stimulation electrode was put in under general anesthesia using the trans-meatal approach. It was fitted through the round-window membrane, which was obscured by lobe fat tissue. We used a round-window electrode and not a promontory electrode because it can be held in a steady position, thus enabling more prolonged testing to be done. The pathway to the concha was done by a polyethylene tube between the bony part and the skin of the external auditory canal. The electrode is 0.02 mm in diameter. These electrodes stayed in place from 1 to 4 days after implantation and allowed the electrical tests to be made. Removal is very easy without the need of further general anesthesia. No tympanic complication was found at the 6-week review.

Electrical testing is objective and subjective:

Electrical stimulation is carried out using Hortmann's Cochlear Nerve Test (CNT):

The objective tests that we performed are the Electrically Evoked Auditory Brain Stem Responses (E-EABRs) and the Electrical Middle Latency Responses (E-MLRs). They were recorded by the Nicolet Pathfinder II.

The subjective tests were of two types.

The *subjective thresholds* were measured when age allowed it. We used Finkenzeller's [1] technique. Subjective hearing electric thresholds and uncomfortable electric thresholds are obtained. The procedure is the same as that used in adults.

When cooperation of the child was difficult due to its age, we tried to perform an *'electrically conditioned orientation reflex'*. Hortmann's CNT induced a current in which pulse width and intensity are increased step by step. We observed the child's reaction during electrical stimulation with the same procedure and technique as used for acoustical stimulation when determining the acoustical hearing threshold of a young deaf child with an acoustically conditioned orientation reflex.

Results

The *E-ABRs and E-MLRs* were recorded in 2 of 6 patients.

We never could distinguish the E-EABRs from the presence of the stimulation artefact. The E-MLRs were recorded easier than the E-ABRs. We observed waves NA at 23 ms and PA at 32.9 ms in the first patient (fig. 1). In the second patient we located waves at 22.2 ms and at 29.9 ms but we think that there were postauricular muscle electrical discharge.

The *subjective electric thresholds* were obtained in 4 of 6 patients (fig. 2–5). The criteria were good for implantation in 3 patients. In the 4th patient the subjective electrical thresholds had very high intensities, and thus we decided that this patient was not suitable for implantation.

It was impossible to get the cooperation of a 2-year-old child. So we performed the 'electrically conditioned orientation reflex'. The responses were modification in behavior, interruption of playing, but not a true orientation to the implanted side. According to the classical acoustical method, the experienced tester interpreted this as manifestation of auditory perception.

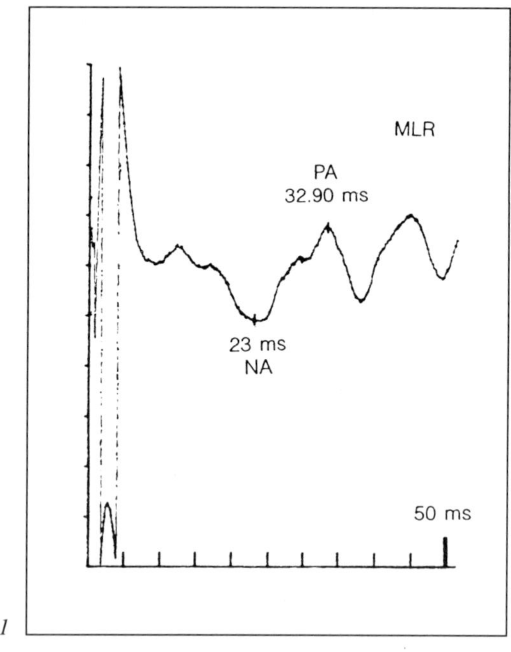

Fig. 1. E-MLRs in a 6-year-old child.
Fig. 2. Subjective thresholds in a 14-year-old child.
Fig. 3. Subjective thresholds in a 6-year-old child.
Fig. 4. Subjective thresholds in a 10-year-old child.
Fig. 5. Subjective thresholds in a 15-year-old child.

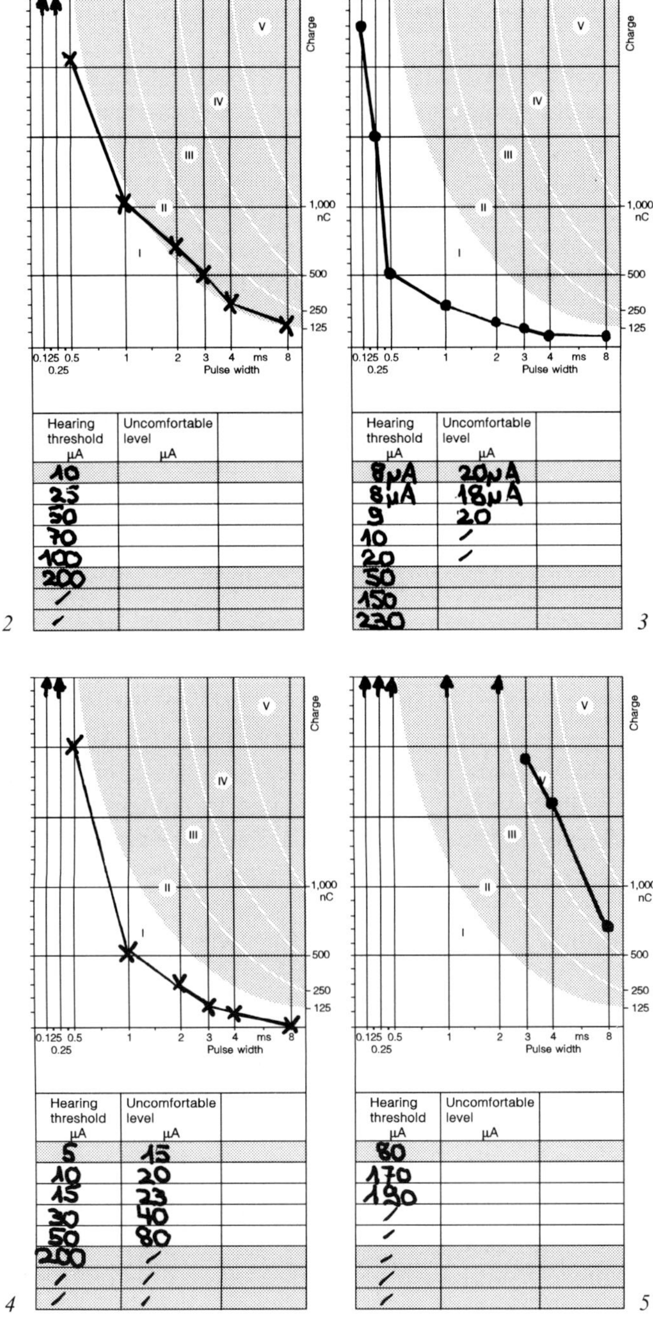
V
IV
III
II
I
Charge
1,000 nC
500
250
125
0.125 0.5
0.25
1
2
3
4
ms
8
Pulse width
Hearing threshold µA
Uncomfortable level µA
10
25
50
70
100
200
8µA 20µA
8µA 18µA
9 20
10
20
50
150
230
5 15
10 20
15 23
30 40
50 80
200
80
170
190

2 3 4 5

This 2-year-old child was implanted; the only proof being that of the 'electrically conditioned orientation reflex', and the preliminary results during the first months of the rehabilitation were good with speech perception and the beginning of linguistic production. Two other children were implanted according to good criterion with Hortmann's CNT and/or recording of E-MLRs. All these children were implanted with the nucleus device.

The 3 other children were not given an implant: one because of high subjective thresholds, one because of psychological problems, and the last because of psychological problems in the mother.

Discussion

In children, the operative technique for the implantation of a temporary electrode is easy. But it needs to be performed under general anesthesia, which is the second one after the tomodensitometry. Thanks to this electrode we can perform some tests which are adjusted to the age of the patient. For us it is very important to get all the information about the ability of the nerve fibers to be excited. Techniques such as E-EABRs are difficult to realise because of the presence of the stimulation artefact. In our experience, E-MLRs are easier to obtain than the E-EABRs. Some authors have described these methods for testing the ability of the remaining nervous fibers to be electrically excited in implant candidates [2–4], or in cochlear implant subjects [5]. The subjective electrical thresholds with Hortmann's CNT can't be reached in very young patients. We have the possibility of getting a subjective response with a conditioned orientation reflex which can be done with an electrical stimulation.

This 'electrically conditioned orientation reflex' is useful but needs the cooperation of a tester who has experience with the acoustical technique.

References

1 Finkenzeller P: Objektive Bewertung elektrischer Stimulation der Hörnerven; in Lehnardt E, Hirshorn MS (eds): Cochlear Implant. Springer, Berlin, 1987, pp 31–36.

2 Banfai P, Karczag A, Kubik S, Luers P, Surth W: Extra-cochlear sixteen-channel electrode system. Otolaryngol Clin North Am 1986;19:371–408.
3 Brightwell A, Rothera M, Conway M, Graham J: Evaluation of the status of the auditory nerve: Psychophysical tests and ABR; in Schindler RA, Merzenic MM (eds): New York, Raven Press, 1985, pp 343–349.
4 Kileny P, Kemick JL: Electrically evoked middle-latency auditory potentials in cochlear implant candidates. Arch Otolaryngol Head Neck Surg 1986;113:1072–1077.
5 Miyamoto RT: Electrically evoked potentials in cochlear implant subjects. Laryngoscope 1986;96:178–185.

E. Truy, MD, Service d'Oto-Rhino-Laryngologie, Hôpital Edouard-Herriot,
5, place d'Arsonval, F–69437 Lyon (France)

Fraysse B, Deguine O (eds): Cochlear Implants: New Perspectives.
Adv Otorhinolaryngol. Basel, Karger, 1993, vol 48, pp 120–124

Brain Stem Evoked Responses by Intracochlear Electric Stimulation

A. Robier, Y. Lescao, P. Beutter

Service ORL, CHU Bretonneau, Tours, France

In the field of cochlear implant assessment, the brain stem response (EABR) and the middle latency evoked response (EMLR) to electric stimulation of the auditory nerve techniques have been developed in the last two decades and are still controversial subjects of debate. Authors as Smith and Simmon [1] for the first technique and Jyung et al. [2] for the second have studied those potentials in animals and described a clear correlation between the reliability of the waves, the slope of the input-output function, and the integrity of the eighth nerve. For Stypulkovski et al. [3], the EABR magnitude and the growth of the magnitude are not related to cochlear pathology but ‘reflect the status of the central auditory pathway rather than the periphery’. The authors stressed that in humans the magnitude of the EABR is smaller making analysis of the data problematic. According to Pellizzone et al. [4] EABR in humans could still give some indication of the status of surviving nerve endings but insist on the necessity of applying the stimulus as close as possible to the surviving nerve population with a monopolar electrode placed as deep as possible in the cochlea.

In this study, developed in humans, we have used the opportunity given by patients implanted with the Ineraid device to compare the EABR elicited before operation with the promontory stimulation and postoperatively on the apical electrode of the electrode array.

Methods

Subjects

Subjects were 6 adults, 3 women, 3 men, ages 42–62 years, with audiometric threshold through 4,000 Hz of less than 90 dB HL. Of the 6 subjects, 3 were deafened by meningitis, 1 by otosclerosis, 1 by ototoxics, and 1 by an unknown aetiology: the duration of profound deafness ranged from 2 years for 4 subjects to 10 and 15 years for the other 2.

Recording and Stimulation

Responses were obtained using silver disk electrodes between the vertex-to-contralateral mastroid with the ground electrode on the forehead. The impedances were less than 3 kΩ. The electrical activity was collected with a commercial instrument (Nicolet CA 1000) with the amplifier set for a band pass of 150–3,000 Hz, and the gain set to 100,000 Hz. The automatic artifact rejection feature of the software was used to exclude electrical activity exceeding ± 10 μV.

A recording window of 10 ms was used with intracochlear stimulation, and of 20 ms with the promontory stimulation.

All testing was done in a single-walled, sound-attenuating test chamber while the subject relaxed in a comfortable reclining chair.

Stimuli were delivered by a commercial instrument (Hortmann Cochlear Nerve Tester) and presented to a transtympanic needle electrode in the first session and to the apical intracochlear electrode of the Ineraid after implantation. Stimuli were presented using alternated electric pulses at a repetition rate of 11.1/s. The pulse width was set to 0.25 or 0.50 ms for the intracochlear stimulation and to 1 or 2 ms for the promontory stimulation, the intensity to 70% of the uncomfortable level and to the electric threshold. A special trigger unit drives a pre-amp to cancel the stimulus electric artefact.

Results

Promontory Stimulation

The data were collected with a promontory stimulation on a transtympanic electrode and all the patients showed that some responses could only be recorded with a 1- or 2-ms pulse width in a 20-ms window. The reliability of the responses is poor and the waves are obscured by a wide stimulus artefact. In the majority of patients only one wave could really be described.

Intracochlear Stimulation

EABR obtained on profoundly deaf subjects implanted with an Ineraid implant showed a good reliability. At 75 μA with a 0.5-ms electric pulse width, the EABR waveform is reliable with three waves labelled: II, III, V. In several patients, wave II is obscured by the electric artefact and in some

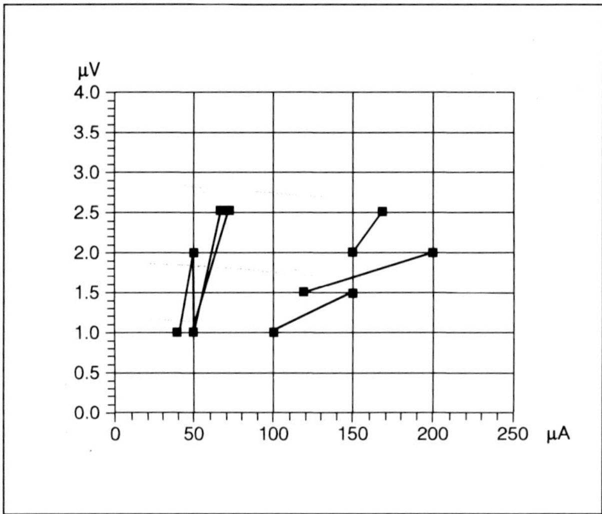

Fig. 1. EABR wave V input-output function for 6 patients with an intracochlear stimulation.

patients wave V is the only response recorded. The latency of responses III and V recorded at 70% of the uncomfortable level was consistent with the literature. In all subjects, as the intensity of the stimulus decreases the latency of each wave increases.

The amplitude of response V has been studied at the maximum stimulus intensity and at the threshold level and the input-output function is shown in figure 1. The slope value is obtained by plotting a line between the threshold and the maximum point. In 3 patients with a low threshold the slope value varies from 0.70 to 0.75. One patient has an higher threshold and a slope value of 0.50. Two patients also have an elevation of the threshold and a low slope value.

All 6 patients underwent various speech and language testings and particularly a French disyllabic word with context test. Without lipreading, the performance of the subjects varies from 0 to 70% recognition.

Regression analysis to compare slope and performance of the patient's implant alone, revealed a significant relationship at the $p < 0.005$ level, with a coefficient of correlation of 0.9 and a coefficient of determination of 80%.

Discussion

The first result to emerge from this study is the demonstration that EABR are difficult to elicit with a promontory stimulation. Pelizzone et al. [4] demonstrated that EABR responses were of poor reliability and of lower amplitude when the stimulation is presented to a promontory electrode or even to a round window electrode than at an apical one. They suggest that for a round window electrode a current at least five times higher is needed to obtain a gradient comparable to intracochlear stimulation. In this condition, as the magnitude of the EABR is also smaller in humans than in animals, the stimulus artefact amplitude obscures the response and the use of a deep intracochlear electrode is quite inevitable.

When an intracochlear electrode is stimulated, the vertex-positive peaks of the EABR are consistent with the waves already reported in humans. The latencies of the waveform in this study seem to be delayed by 0.5 ms, this could be explained by the difficult to assume triggering point; in this respect, the latencies are in good agreement with the data reported in the literature. As discussed by Stypulkowski et al. [3], wave I directly reflects that the activity of the auditory nerve remnants is absent in the EABR, and response II to V reflect the activity of more central structures.

The elevation of the EABR threshold is the second issue under discussion and for Smith and Simmons [1], an elevation in the EABR threshold only occurred in ears with 5% or less ganglion cells in the lower basal turn. The elevation of the threshold in some patients could also be explained by osseous lesions of the modiolus reducing the flow of current toward the ganglion cell bodies.

The input-output function of EABR wave V has been studied in animals. It has been observed that the growth of the EABR was sensitive to the modification in the population of excitable neural elements. Smith and Simmons [1] had demonstrated that even if as little as 5% or less ganglion cells produce an EABR the slope of the EABR input-output function was related to the spiral ganglion cell losses. In the same way, Juyng et al. [2], in an EMLR study, have shown that the slope of the input-output function reflects the number of surviving spiral ganglion cells. He also stated that the EMLR threshold does not depend on the ganglion cell population.

In this study, for 3 patients a low electric threshold is associated with steep slopes of the EABR input-output function and excellent postimplant results. On the contrary, 2 patients an elevation of the electric threshold is associated with a decline of the slope and poor results without lipreading. In one patient deafened by meningitis, the association of the elevation of the threshold to the steepness of the slope could possibly reflect the existence of a functional surviving population and the reduction of the flow of current.

Conclusion

Even if EABR could represent an interesting clinical tool, technical problems like position of the electrode and type of electric stimulus remain and need to be solved to improve the waveform recording. In our opinion, at present the technique is still limited to a rather experimental field.

References

1 Smith L, Simmons F: Estimating eight nerve survival by electric stimulation. Ann Otol Rhinol Laryngol 1983;92:19–23.
2 Jyung RW, Miller JM, Cannon SC: Evaluation of eighth nerve integrity by the electrically evoked middle latency response. Otolaryngol Head Neck Surg 1989;101: 670–682.
3 Stypulkowki PH, van den Hornert C, Kvistad SD: Electrophysiologic evaluation of the cochlear implant patient. Otolaryngol Clin North Am 1986;19:249–257.
4 Pelizzone M, Kasper A, Montandon P: Electrically evoked responses in cochlear implant patients. Audiology 1989;28:230–238.
5 Kasper A, Pelizzone M, Montandon P: Intracochlear potential distribution with intracochlear and extracochlear electrical stimulation in humans. Ann Otol Rhinol Laryngol 1991;100:812–816.

Prof. A. Robier, Service ORL, CHU Bretonneau, Boulevard Tonnelé,
F–37044 Tours (France)

Fraysse B, Deguine O (eds): Cochlear Implants: New Perspectives.
Adv Otorhinolaryngol. Basel, Karger, 1993, vol 48, pp 125–129

Auditory Brain Stem Response Evoked by Electrical Stimulation with a Cochlear Implant

Catherine D. Brown[a], *Trisha Antognelli*[b], *William P.R. Gibson*[c]

[a] Children's Cochlear Implant Centre, Naremburn, NSW;
[b] Cochlear Pty. Ltd., Lane Cove, NSW;
[c] Department of Surgery, Sydney University, Sydney, Australia

Recent research has demonstrated the benefits obtained by children who have received the Nucleus 22 channel cochlear implant [1–3]. Benefits obtained from a cochlear implant depend upon many factors [4], but initially, perhaps the most important consideration is the establishment of optimum signal for the child which is comfortable and not unpleasant in any way.

The relationship of patients' EABR to their behavioural responses to electrical stimulation has been investigated by several research groups [5–8]. In this study, we compare the EABR wave V threshold with behaviour thresholds and comfort levels for electrical stimulation once a stable program has been established which is typically 6 months after initial stimulation.

Methods

Subjects

Twenty-six patients were tested 4 weeks postoperatively at the Children's Hospital, Camperdown, NSW. The children were admitted as day-stay patients. Fourteen of the children have congenital hearing losses and 12 have acquired losses. All of the children with acquired hearing loss were deafened by meningitis. The age of the children ranged from 2 years 2 months to 12 years at the time of testing.

Equipment

The Nucleus cochlear implant receiver/stimulator and 22 channel electrode array had been implanted in all of the children in this study. The internal device was activated by the Nucleus WSP III speech processor via the Nucleus speech processor interface (SPI).

The SPI was connected to a Sanyo personal computer which had been modified to run the Diagnostic and Programming Software (DPU version 4.14) supplied by Cochlear Pty. Ltd.

The stimuli used were biphasic square pulses with a 204 μs pulse width. The stimulus duration was set to 1,000 milliseconds (ms) with an inter-stimulus wait time of 1 ms. The repetition rate was 10 or 11 pulses per second. The stimuli were generated by the SPI and delivered to the patient via the WSP headset. A triggering device linked the WSP to the recording set up. Latencies were measured from the WSP trigger time.

Eight subcutaneous recording electrodes were placed at the vertex (positive) and contralateral earlobe (reference) with four electrodes at the forehead (ground). These 8 electrodes were paired to produce 4 recording channels. The 4 signals were first passed through 4 independent low pass filters to reduce the RF artefact [9] and then through 4 independent pre-amplifiers and on to a Medelec ER94a pre-amplifier. The band-pass filter settings of the Medelec ER94a were 1 Hz to 6 kHz. Analysis time was 10 ms and 256–512 stimuli were averaged per recording. These 4 recordings were averaged producing a single record.

Procedure

Recording sessions typically lasted 1–2 h. The patients were anaesthetised and a muscle relaxant was administered for the duration of the recording session in order to prevent skeletal muscle activity from interfering with the EABR recordings.

EABR thresholds were obtained on 5–6 electrodes E20, E15, E11, E3, and E1. If E1 had been placed outside close to the round window, a response typically could not be obtained. A check of the remaining electrodes would then be carried out at current level 192 to ensure the untested electrodes were functional.

Behavioural thresholds (T levels) and maximum comfort levels (C levels) were taken from the children's MAPs obtained approximately 6 months after surgery. As all the children wear the mini speech processor (MSP) and are programmed using 'stimulus levels' and the EABR results were obtained with a Wearable Speech Processor (WSP) utilising 'current levels' as a measure of the stimulus, the levels obtained have all been converted to a measure of charge per phase in nanocoulombs (nC) using conversion tables supplied by Cochlear Pty. Ltd.

Results

Morphology

The morphology of the waveforms recorded from patients with congenital hearing loss differed from those recorded from patients with hearing loss acquried as a result of meningitis. Typically, four distinct waves were observed in the meningitic patients. In the congenital patients, the third and fourth waves were combined, forming a broader, less distinct

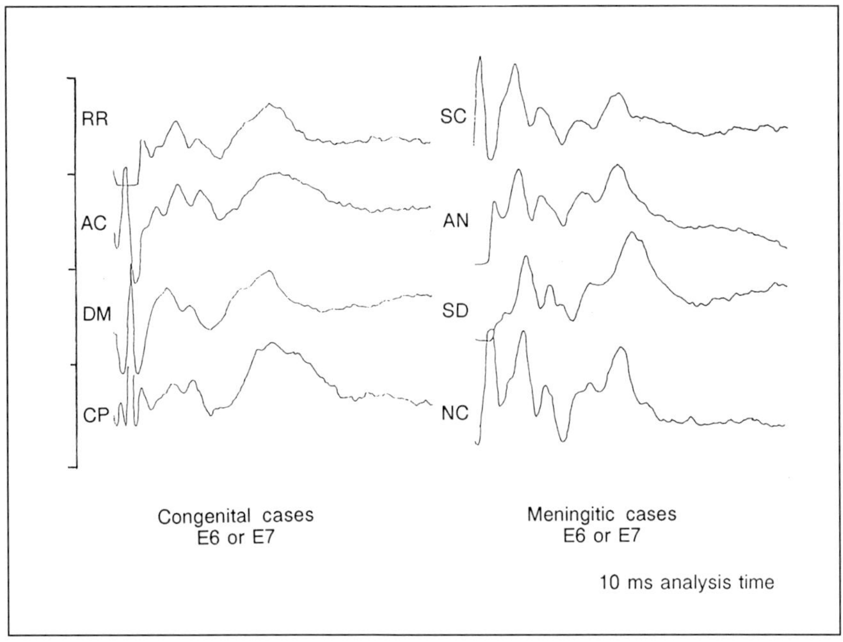

Fig. 1. Evoked potentials obtained from 4 congenitally hearing impaired children and 4 children deafened by meningitis demonstrating the difference in the morphology of the waveforms.

waveform. Typical waveforms from 4 children with a congenital hearing loss and 4 with an acquired hearing loss are shown in figure 1.

The relationship between the EABR wave V threshold obtained for electrodes 20, 11 and 3 for each group and the behavioural thresholds and comfort levels obtained approximately 6 months after the initial programming sessions (or when a stable, reliable MAP had been obtained) were examined. The mean EABR thresholds were higher than the mean behavioural thresholds for both the congenitally hearing impaired subjects and the subjects with acquired hearing loss. The mean behavioural comfort levels showed a closer relationship to the mean EABR thresholds overall. However, a Pearson correlation matrix revealed very poor correlation between the EABR thresholds and either the behavioural C levels or T levels for all electrodes in both groups. The groups were combined but there was still poor correlation with the EABR thresholds.

Conclusions

Despite the fact that no overall relationship between the objective and subjective measurements has been established, the EABR results have been found to be a useful clinical tool at the Children's Cochlear Implant Centre (NSW). These results provide an indication of the integrity of the auditory pathway and of possible malfunctioning electrodes. Any electrodes which give anomalous results can thus be avoided until an implant integrity test can be carried out.

The results of the EABR are utilised during the initial programming of the Nucleus 22 channel cochlear implant for young children who are unable to produce reliable responses to auditory stimuli. If interpreted with caution, the EABR thresholds can be used as a guide for estimating the initial maximum comfort levels. The clinician can be confident that if these levels are not exceeded, then the child should not be subjected to a level of sound that is uncomfortable. If the thresholds are set at an arbitrary level below the EABR thresholds when behavioural thresholds cannot be obtained, the MAP thus obtained should provide the child with an auditory stimulus. Once the child has become accustomed to sound, then training in stimulus/response techniques can be started and accurate thresholds established.

Therefore, with EABR results, clinic personnel can be confident that the initial program of threshold and comfort levels provided to the child is not uncomfortable and that the child can hear a signal which can be refined and perfected as the child matures. This allows more confident counselling of the parents in how to manage their child during the initial stages of programming, thereby ensuring a smoother transition into the world of sound.

References

1 Staller SJ, Beiter AL, Brimacombe JA, Mecklenbury DJ, Arndt P: Pediatric performance with the Nucleus 22-channel cochlear implant system. Am J Otol 1991;12: 126–136.

2 Dowell RC, Dawson PW, Dettman SJ, Shepherd RK, Whitford LA, Seligman PM, Clark GM: Mutlichannel cochlear implantation in children: A summary of current work at the University of Melbourne. Am J Otol 1991;12:137–143.

3 Osberger MJ, Robbins AM, Miyamoto RT, Berry SW, Myres WA, Kessler KS, Pope ML: Speech perception abilities of children with cochlear implants, tactile aids, or hearing aids. Am J Otol 1991;12:105–115.

4 Brown CD, Yaremko R: Special considerations of cochler implants in children. Aust J Hum Commun Dis 1991;19:25–30.

5 Shallop JK, Beiter AL, Goin DW, Mischke RE: Electrically evoked auditory brain stem responses (EABR) and middle latency responses (EMLR) obtained from patients with the nucleus multichannel cochlear implant. Ear Hear 1990;11:5–15.

6 Abbas PJ, Brown CJ: Electrically evoked auditory brainstem response: Growth of response with current level. Hear Res 1991;51:123–138.

7 Miyamoto RT, Brown DD: Electrically evoked brainstem responses in cochlear implant recipients. Otol Head Neck Surg 1987;96:34–38.

8 Starr A, Brackmann DE: Brain stem potentials evoked by electrical stimulation of the cochlea in human subjects. Ann Otol 1979;88:550–556.

9 Game CJA, Thomson DR, Gibson WPR: Measurement of auditory brainstem responses evoked by electrical stimulation with a cochlear implant. Br J Audiol 1990;24:145–149.

Catherine Brown, MA (Aud.), Children's Cochlear Implant Centre,
246a Willoughby Road, Naremburn, NSW 2065 (Australia)

Fraysse B, Deguine O (eds): Cochlear Implants: New Perspectives.
Adv Otorhinolaryngol. Basel, Karger, 1993, vol 48, pp 130–135

Electrical Brain Stem Responses in Cochlear Implant Patients

Bent Almqvist, Sten Harris, Karl-Erik Jönsson

Department of Audiology, University Hospital, Lund, Sweden

Electrical brain stem responses, E-ABR, can be used in predicting T levels and in electrode function tests in cochlear implant patients [1]. The purpose of this paper is to present a method specifically designed to record E-ABR through the Nucleus implant.

Material and Methods

Subjects

Thirteen patients implanted with the Nucleus mini 22 system were included in the study. Ten patients have been tested in a rate/threshold study. Five patients were selected for more extensive E-ABR measurements including both threshold and stimulus pulse studies.

Equipment

The E-ABR response from the Nucleus implant measured with a standard ABR preamplifier gives a large artefact generated by the stimulus pulse and the 2.5-MHz radio signal. In order to avoid this problem we have made the following modifications in our equipment. A low-pass radio filter is used to prevent the radio signal to interfere [2]. The op amplifiers are fast in order to shorten the recovery time so the amplifier does not get saturated by the stimulus. Finally, a somewhat wider analog filter is used to give the possibility to study the stimulus pulses.

To minimize the size of the equipment and to avoid two computers, a 2.5-MHz transmitter has been built. The transmitter works at a rate of 17 Hz.

The software gives possibilities for alternating stimulation. When stimulating BP+1 the artefact starts with a positive pulse. When stimulating the same electrodes in the BP–1

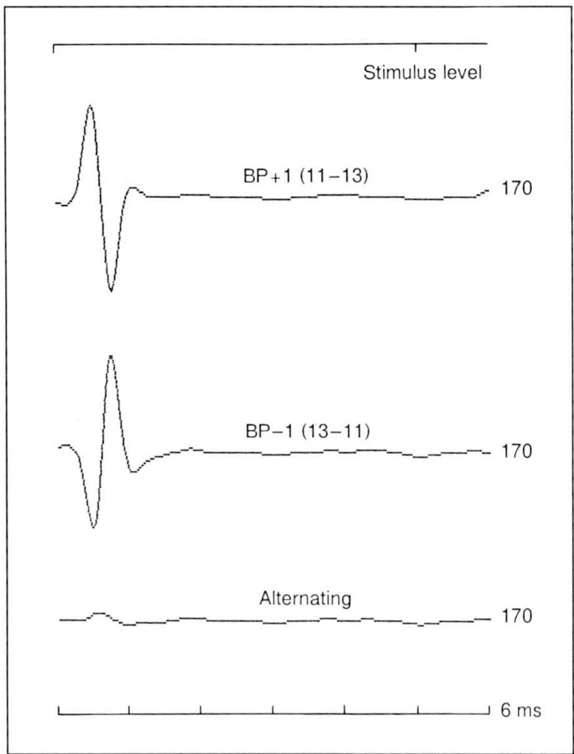

Fig. 1. Stimulus artefacts from BP+1 and BP–1 mode on the same two electrodes. The artefact is reduced by alternating between these two modes.

mode the artifact conversingly starts with a negative pulse. The effect of alternating between these stimulus modes can be seen in figure 1. The software has also been developed to give us possibilities to work with 8 levels or 8 electrodes in parallel. Digital filtering can be applied on the collected data. We have used a linear phase filter.

The chosen trigger point is the start of 'phase 1'. This gives us possibilities to work with different stimulus levels without considering pulse-length/latency problems.

Results

In our group of 13 patients we got nice registrations in 9 cases, detectable E-ABRs in 3 cases, and no responses in one case.

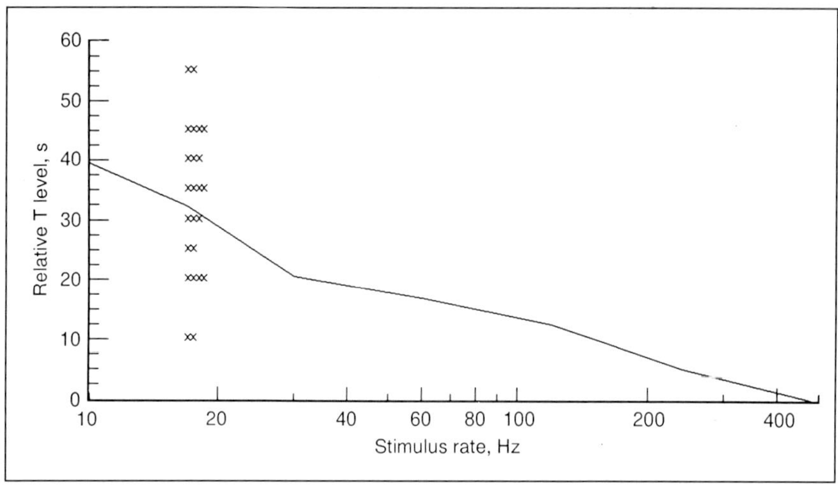

Fig. 2. Threshold shift as function of stimulus rate. Normalized at 480 Hz. The solid line represents the mean value. The individual results are plotted for the 17-Hz rate.

Threshold Difference

In order to determine the differences between subjective thresholds for various stimulus rates 10 patients were tested for seven different rates between 10 and 480 stimuli/s (fig. 2). All measurements were performed at the stimulus level and the thresholds were normalized at the 480 rate. The results show great variations. The individual results for 17 stimuli/s are shown. The mean value difference between 17 and 480 Hz is 32 stimulus levels.

E-ABR Threshold

Figure 3 shows an example of an E-ABR registration from one of the 5 investigated patients. The stimulus artefact is followed by Jewett waves II to V. Figure 3 also presents the registered E-ABR latencies for waves II to V as measured 50 stimulus levels above the 17-Hz subjective T level. The difference between the E-ABR threshold and the 17-Hz subjective T level was found to be 17 stimulus levels with a SD of 7.5. The difference between the E-ABr threshold and the 500-Hz subjective T level was 42 stimulus levels with a SD of 18.

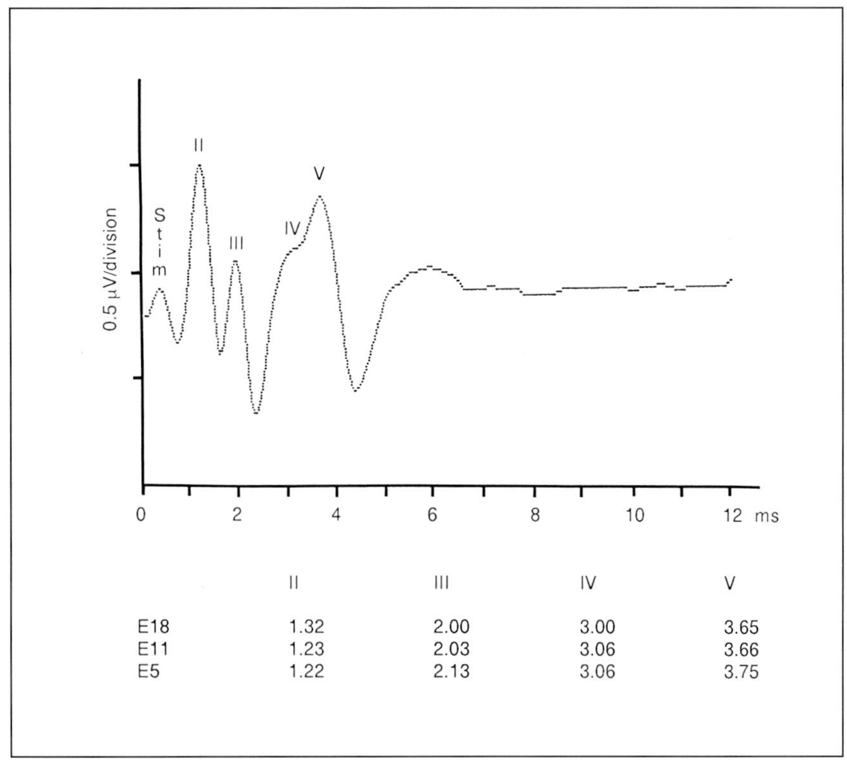

	II	III	IV	V
E18	1.32	2.00	3.00	3.65
E11	1.23	2.03	3.06	3.66
E5	1.22	2.13	3.06	3.75

Fig. 3. A typical E-ABR recording. Mean values for Jewett waves II to V latencies in ms below.

Stimulus Pulses

In figures 4a and 4b, the stimulus pulses from all 22 electrodes are presented in both CG and BP+1 mode. The CG registration in figure 4a shows that all current at the basal end is forced in an apical direction giving rise to a large pulse which starts negative. At the apical end all current is forced in the opposite basal direction giving rise to a large pulse starting positive. In the middle part we have a symmetrical situation with a current flow in both directions with small registered pulses. The BP+1 registration shows low amplitudes in the apical end and larger amplitudes in the basal end.

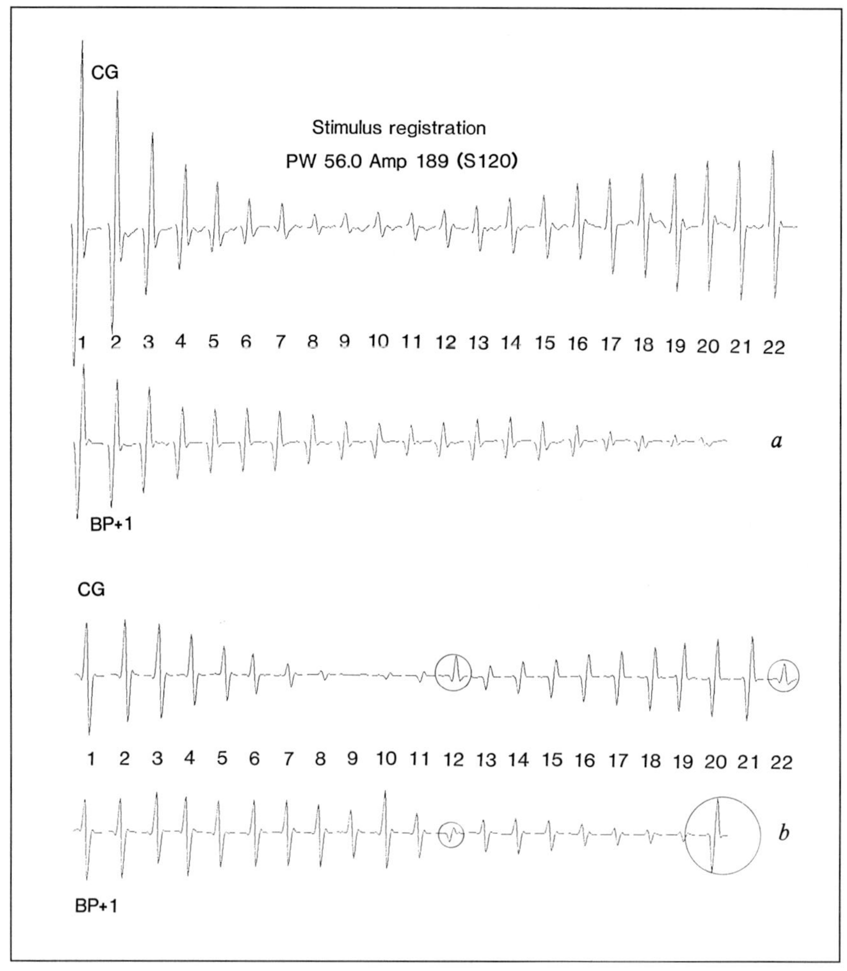

Fig. 4. a Stimulus registration from an implant with all electrodes working correctly. *b* Stimulus registration from an implant with failure on electrodes 12 and 22.

The patient recorded in figure 4b complained of a suddenly developed low pitch for electrode number 12. The CG registration shows different shapes for electrodes 12 and 22. The BP+1 registration gives a low amplitude and opposite polarity for electrode 12. Electrode 20 has opposite phase and a high amplitude.

Discussion

Our E-ABR recordings are very similar to the pattern we are familiar with from the acoustic ABR. The latencies are about 2 ms shorter. Different authors, however, have been using different trigger points [2–4]. This is of importance to have in mind when comparing absolute latency measurements. In our study the absolute E-ABR latencies, 50 stimulus levels above the 17-Hz threshold, is almost the same for the different electrodes. This is contrary to the findings of Allum et al. [3] and Shallop et al. [4], who found differences between the apical and basal electrodes.

Registration of stimulus pulses can be very useful in finding defect electrodes, i.e. open circuits and shorts in the electrode array. The method is fast and takes only about 10 min for a complete test at a rate of 17 Hz.

In summary, E-ABR performed with the described technique has proven to be a valuable method to test the cochlear implant function and to predict T levels.

References

1 Shallop JK, VanDyke L, Goin DW, Mischke RE: Prediction of behavioral thresholds and comfort values for Nucleus 22-channel implant patients from electrical auditory brain stem response test results. Ann Otol Rhinol Laryngol 1991;100:896–898.

2 Game CJA, Thomson DR, Gibson WPR: Measurement of auditory brainstem responses evoked by electrical stimulation with a cochlear implant. Br J Audiol 1990;24:145–149.

3 Allum JH, Shallop JK, Hotz M, Pfaltz CR: Characteristics of electrically evoked 'auditory' brainstem responses elicited with the Nucleus 22-electrode intracochlear implant. Scand Audiol 1990;19:263–267.

4 Shallop JK, Beiter AL, Goin DW, Miscke RE: Electrically evoked auditory brain stem responses (EABR) and middle latency responses (EMLR) obtained from patients with the nucleus multichannel cochlear implant. Ear Hear 1990;11:5–15.

Dr. Sten Harris, Audiology Department, University Hospital,
S–221 85 Lund (Sweden)

Fraysse B, Deguine O (eds): Cochlear Implants: New Perspectives.
Adv Otorhinolaryngol. Basel, Karger, 1993, vol 48, pp 136–141

Application of Intraoperative Recordings of Electrically Evoked ABRs in a Paediatric Cochlear Implant Programme

S.M. Mason[a], *S. Sheppard*[c], *C.W. Garnham*[a], *M.E. Lutman*[d], *G.M. O'Donoghue*[b], *K.P. Gibbin*[b]

on behalf of The Nottingham Paediatric Cochlear Implant Group

[a]Medical Physics Department, [b]Department of Otolaryngology, Queen's Medical Centre; [c]Paediatric Cochlear Implant Group, [d]Institute of Hearing Research, General Hospital, Nottingham, UK

Cochlear implantation is now benefitting an increasing number of profoundly deaf young children who obtain little or no hearing from conventional amplification [1]. Behavioural methods for setting the electrical stimulation parameters for each individual child present a difficult challenge in these young patients when compared to older children and adults. In this situation 'objective' evoked potential methods [2] can play an important role in the assessment. The auditory brain stem response can be evoked electrically (EABR) by a cochlear implant [3–5] and is an appropriate response to record in young children [6]. This technique is therefore potentially very valuable in young children as a means of assessing the functioning of the cochlear implant device.

An intraoperative recording technique for the EABR has been developed for use in the Paediatric Cochlear Implant Programme in Nottingham. EABR measurements are carried out during surgery after implantation of the Nucleus 22 channel electrode array and receiver. Technical aspects and difficulties of the procedure are described including the relationship between the intraoperative EABR characteristics and behavioural threshold (T) levels at the initial stimulation period.

Methodology and Materials

Stimulus Generation

Electrical stimulation by the Nucleus 22 channel implant is controlled by the mini speech processor (MSP) and the dual processor interface (DPI). The DPI is interfaced to an IBM PS2 computer which utilizes the diagnostic and programming software (DPS 6.53). Biphasic electrical pulses are generated in the stimulus mode on a selected channel of the implant device. A 1-second burst of pulses is initiated at a repetition rate of 31 pps. A sufficient number of bursts are generated to complete a recording of the averaged waveform (1,024 or 2,048 sweeps). Common ground (CG) stimulus mode is usually selected when complete insertion of the electrode array has been achieved.

Recording Equipment

A Medelec Mistral evoked potential system is used to acquire the response waveforms and is triggered from the DPI unit. The on-line EEG signal is recorded from surface electrodes positioned at the vertex and contralateral mastoid. A guard electrode is positioned on the forehead. Electrode leads are colour coded for future reference since it is not possible to trace the electrode wires during the surgical procedure. A passive filter network (modified from Game et al. [7]) is placed in-line with the recording electrode leads immediately before the preamplifier in order to reduce the effects of radiofrequency (RF) interference arising from the transcutaneous transmission system. Amplifier sensitivity is set to 10 or 20 μV per division depending on the level of activity on the signal baseline. The on-line EEG signal is filtered with a bandwidth from 100 to 3,000 Hz and signal averaged with a post-stimulus epoch of 10 ms.

Test Procedure

The recording electrodes are securely attached to the scalp immediately after administration of the general anaesthetic and before the patient is prepared for surgery. Collodion glue is used for attachment of the vertex electrode and surgical adhesive tape for other sites. Contact impedances are less than 4k Ω for each electrode.

After implantation of the electrode array and receiver, the transmitter coil/lead is placed in a sterile clear plastic sheath (40 mm × 1 m) and is positioned over the receiver in the wound. EABR measurements are carried out immediately after completion of the measurement of the electrical stapedius reflex thresholds [8]. Response waveforms are recorded with a range of electrical stimulus levels on electrode channels 20, 15, 10 and 5. The stimulus level is changed in steps of 20 units at high suprathreshold levels and in steps of 10 units close to threshold, EABR threshold being estimated to the nearest 5 units by interpolation. This protocol can be completed in about 20–30 min during closure of the wound and suturing of the skin flap, and requires very little additional operating-theatre time.

Subjects

Analysis is presented in 12 children with ages ranging from 2 years 6 months to 9 years. Ten children had a profound hearing loss following meningitis and 2 were congenitally deaf. Complete insertion of the electrode array was achieved in all children except one (17 channels). The EABR threshold was compared to the behavioural threshold (T) level from the first reliable map which was obtained at around 4 weeks after implantation.

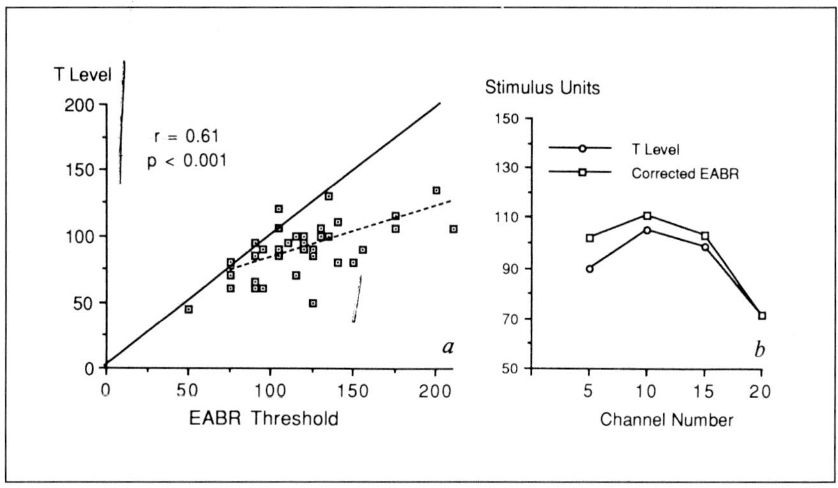

Fig. 1. The relationship between the EABR threshold and subjective T level with respect to (*a*) stimulus threshold and (*b*) electrode channel. The solid line in (*a*) represents equal values and the dotted line the linear regression ($y = 46 + 0.37x$, where y = T level and x = EABR threshold).

Measurement of T level employed a performance test technique using a 250 pps pulse rate stimulus presented as a 1-second burst. The EABR and T level data include 39 threshold measurements with channels 20, 15, 10, and 5 having 12, 11, 9 and 7 measurements, respectively. Early in the study, reliable data could not be recorded on all four channels due to either time constraints or technical difficulties.

Results

The relationships between EABR threshold and subjective T level are illustrated in figure 1. In general, the EABR threshold, recorded with a pulse rate of 31 pps, is slightly less sensitive than the 250-pps pulse rate T level, with group mean (SD) measurements for the 39 thresholds of 119 (33) and 90 (20) stimulus units, respectively. If 30 stimulus units is subtracted from each of the EABR thresholds as a correction factor, then 82% are within 30 stimulus units of the T level.

The performance of the EABR in predicting the T level is dependent on the stimulus level of the threshold and the electrode channel. The scatterplot of the EABR thresholds and T levels (fig. 1a) demonstrates that the EABR becomes progressively less sensitive as a predictor of T level with increased stimulus threshold. The sensitivity of the EABR threshold is also related to the electrode channel. In figure 1b, the mean EABR threshold for channel 20 has been equated to the T level using a correction factor of 24 stimulus units. This same correction factor has then been applied to all the individual EABR thresholds of the other channels. The result clearly demonstrates a progressive increase in divergence between the EABR threshold and T level at the more basal electrode sites. The configuration of the EABR thresholds and T levels across the four electrode channels shows the typical 'bell-shape' often associated with common ground stimulation.

Discussion

The quality of the recording of the intraoperative EABR waveform is dependent on a number of factors such as the use of optimum data collection parameters, a low level of noise and interference on the signal baseline, and how effectively the surviving auditory nerve fibres are being stimulated. The problem of stimulus-related artefacts on the recording signal is exacerbated with electrical stimulation in contrast to an acoustical stimulus. These artefacts arise from the RF transmitter signal and the electrical stimulus. The RF component of the artefact is effectively removed by the RF filter. The level of contamination of the waveforms with the electrical stimulus artefact is variable between test sessions, being dependent to some extent on the contact impedance of the recording electrodes. The artefact, however, only occasionally interferes with the response waveform with stimulus levels above 200 units.

Characteristics of the EABR waveform are slightly different to those recorded for the acoustical ABR. Absolute latency of the electrical evoked components are shorter with wave eV arising at about 4.0–4.5 ms. There is only a small increase in latency with reduction in stimulus level in contrast to the acoustical ABR. These findings are consistent with the lack of a cochlear travelling wave as a component of the process. The low frequency signal components associated with wave V and SN10 in the acoustic ABR waveform (below 100 Hz) are absent in the EABR. There is therefore no advantage in employing a signal filter with a 20- or 30-Hz low frequency cut-off since an improvement of the response to noise amplitude ratio will not be achieved. A 100-Hz high pass filter has therefore been adopted.

Amplitude of the wave eV component of the EABR is very small close-to-threshold (typically 50 nV). A good quality signal baseline, combined with signal averaging of 2,000 sweeps with appropriate replication, is required in order to achieve reliable identification of the response waveform and good sensitivity of the EABR threshold.

Analysis of the EABR threshold with respect to the T level shows that, with the introduction of an appropriate correction factor, there is valuable agreement between the two measures. The ability of the EABR to predict the T level will be enhanced when the effects of absolute stimulus threshold and electrode channel are taken into consideration. More extensive datasets will help to define these correction factors more accurately. A significant proportion of the apparent lack of sensitivity of the EABR with respect to the T level arises as a result of the different pulse rates employed for each measurement. The pulse rate used for recording the EABR is relatively slow (31 pps) compared to the 250 pps usually employed for measurement of the T level. This will introduce a difference in sensitivity between the two measurements due to the effects of temporal integration in the central auditory pathways. Larger discrepancies between the EABR threshold and T level, due to an apparent lack of sensitivity of the EABR, have been reported by Shallop et al. [9]. However, in their study the Nucleus WSPIII speech processor was employed along with different stimulus and recording parameters for the EABR.

This study has demonstrated the value of intraoperative EABR measurements in young children. These recordings have already proved very valuable for several children in the implant programme. Behavioural assessment was so difficult to initiate for 2 of the children during the initial test session that the T level settings were strongly influenced by the EABR thresholds until a more accurate and reliable assessment could be determined subjectively.

Conclusion

Intraoperative measurement of the EABR is a viable technique in young children receiving cochlear implants and should be one of the tools routinely available in a paediatric cochlear implant programme. It provides information about the functioning of the electrode array, indicating suitable levels of electrical stimulation for sensation of the stimulus in the initial behavioural tuning-in session.

Acknowledgements

The authors are grateful for financial support from the Hearing Research Trust. Appreciation is also expressed to the technical staff of the Evoked Potentials Clinic in the Medical Physics Department.

References

1 Staller SJ: Multichannel cochlear implants in children. Ear Hear 1991;12(suppl).
2 Kileny PR: Use of electrophysiologic measures in the management of children with cochlear implants: Brainstem, middle latency, and cognitive (P300) responses. Am J Otol 1991;12(suppl):37–42.
3 Miyamoto RT: Electrically evoked potentials in cochlear implants. Laryngoscope 1986;96:178–185.
4 Abbas PJ, Brown CJ: Electrically evoked brainstem potentials in cochlear implant patients with multi-electrode stimulation. Hear Res 1988;36:153–162.
5 Allum JHJ, Shallop JK, Hotz M, Pfaltz CR: Characteristics of electrically evoked 'auditory' brainstem responses elicited with the Nucleus 22-electrode intracochlear implant. Scand Audiol 1990;19:263–267.
6 Jacobson JT: The Auditory Brainstem Response. San Diego, College-Hill Press, 1985.
7 Game CJA, Thomson DR, Gibson WPR: Measurement of auditory brainstem responses evoked by electrical stimulation with a cochlear implant. Br J Audiol 1990;24:145–149.
8 Sheppard S, Mason SM, Lutman ME, Gibbin KP, O'Donoghue GM: Intraoperative electrical stapedial reflex measurements in young children receiving cochlear implants. Ear Hear 1993; in preparation.
9 Shallop JK, VanDyke L, Goin DW, Mischke RE: Prediction of behavioural threshold and comfort values for Nucleus 22-channel implant patients from electrical auditory brain stem response test results. Ann Otol Rhinol Laryngol 1991;100:896–898.

S.M. Mason, PhD, Consultant Medical Physicist, Medical Physics Department, Queen's Medical Centre, Nottingham NG7 2UH (UK)

Fraysse B, Deguine O (eds): Cochlear Implants: New Perspectives.
Adv Otorhinolaryngol. Basel, Karger, 1993, vol 48, pp 142–145

Predictive Factors in Cochlear Implant Surgery

O. Deguine[a], *B. Fraysse*[a], *A. Uziel*[b], *N. Cochard*[a],
F. Reuillard-Artières[b], *J.P. Piron*[b], *M. Mondain*[b]

[a]CHU Purpan, Service ORL, Toulouse;
[b]CHU Saint-Charles, Service ORL, Montpellier, France

The success of cochlear implantation depends on preoperative, preoperative and postoperative factors. In a series of 50 patients implanted with the Nucleus 22 system, the authors analyze the prognostic values of different factors such as age of onset of deafness, duration of auditory deprivation, age of implantation, promontory test stimulation, cochlear ossification, length of electrode insertion, location of electrode (scala tympani/scala vestibuli), etiology of deafness, number of active electrodes, and MAP dynamic range. The patients are distributed into three groups according to their speech discrimination in open set conditions.

Material and Methods

Seventy-seven cochlear implantations have been performed in Toulouse and Montpellier. For this study, we considered the 50 patients implanted with a Nucleus device, which was used for the first time in France, in Toulouse, in 1987. Table 1 shows the ages at the time of implantation, and table 2 describes the etiologies of deafness.

Fourteen patients were deaf prelingually and 36 patients postlingually. At the time of surgery, we encountered a normal cochlea in 64% of the cases, partial ossification ($\leq$8 mm) in 30% of the cases, and total ossification ($>$8 mm) in 6% of the cases. In the case of total ossification, we performed a partial insertion in 2 cases, and a total insertion through the scala vestibuli in 1 case.

Patients were evaluated without lipreading, with open set sentences without context. Children were evaluated with a visual support (pictures). The patients were divided into three groups: Group I (excellent): discrimination $\geq$60% (or acquisition of language for children). Group II (moderate): discrimination $<$60%. Group III (poor): no discrimination. The clinical results are given in table 3; they were available for 45 patients (follow-up $\geq$2 months).

Table 1. Age at surgery

Age	n
3–10	14
10–20	4
20–30	5
30–40	8
40–50	8
50–60	5
60–70	4
70–80	2

Table 2. Etiology of deafness

Etiology	Patients	
	n	%
Meningitis	11	22
Congenital	8	16
Unknown	6	12
Traumatic	6	12
Chronic otitis	4	8
Mumps	4	8
Otosclerosis	4	8
Systemic disease	4	8
Ototoxic	2	4
Menière's disease	1	2

Table 3. Clinical results

	Group I	Group II	Group III
Adults	14	6	8
Children	5	6	6
Total (%)	19 (42)	12 (27)	14 (31)

Table 4. Repartition of pre- and postlingual

	Group I		Group II		Group III	
	n	%	n	%	n	%
Postlingual	18	55	7	21	8	24
Prelingual	1	8	5	42	6	50
Total	19	42	12	27	14	31

Chi-square = 7.70, p = 0.02.

Predictive factors were evaluated with statistical software (Statview II) on a Macintosh II Ci PC. We used nonparametric tests (Kruskall-Wallis, and Anova; significance 95% – factorial experiments). Predictive factors were calculated on the global population, then separately on the pre- and postlingual populations. To define the profile of the 'excellent implant user', we considered predictive factors of group I vs. group II vs. group III and group I vs. group II + III.

Results

In the total population, we found 5 significant factors characterizing the 'excellent patient': (1) postlingual deafness; (2) short duration of auditory deprivation; (3) high promontory test dynamic; (4) low proportion of inactivated electrodes; (5) high MAP dynamic range (tables 4, 5). Etiology of deafness, sudden versus progressive onset of deafness, and presence of partial cochlear ossification were not significant factors in this study.

Conclusion

It was possible to point out: (a) Preoperative significant predictive factors: postlingual vs. prelingual deafness, duration of auditory deprivation, and the promontory test dynamic (adults). (b) Peroperative significant predictive factors in the postlingual population: length of electrode insertion. (c) Postoperative significant predictive factors: proportion of inactivated electrodes, and the MAP dynamic range.

Table 5. Predictive factors

	Group	n	Mean	SD	SE	Anova	F test
Duration of auditory deprivation	I	19	3.73	4.09	0.93	I vs. III	
	II	12	10.18	12.59	3.63	Fisher PLSD = 7.58*	p = 0.05
	III	14	12.82	14.50	3.87		
Promontory test dynamic	I	15	10.55	7.07	1.82	I vs. II + III	
	II + III	16	6.47	3.23	0.80	Fisher PLSD = 3.99*	
						Scheffe F test = 4.37*	p = 0.04
Proportion inactivated electrodes	I	18	0.008	0.023	0.006	I vs. III	
	II	12	0.076	0.112	0.032	Fisher PLSD = 0.083*	p = 0.003
	III	14	0.156	0.175	0.047	Scheffe F test = 6.552*	
MAP dynamic range	I	18	70.16	29.75	7.01	I vs. II + III	
	II + III	26	50.15	30.00	5.88	Fisher PLSD = 18.50*	p = 0.03
						Scheffe F test = 4.46*	
Length of electrode insertion (postlingual)	I	18	21.79	1.90	0.44	I vs. II + III	
	II + III	15	19.86	3.16	0.81	Fisher PLSD = 1.81*	p = 0.03
						Scheffe F test = 4.70*	

* Significant at 95%.

We could not evaluate the influence of the duration of rehabilitation or of training with the cochlear implant, although they are probably two of the main factors contributing to the success of cochlear implantation. Further follow-up is needed to evaluate the influence of type and duration of rehabilitation, and the results in prelingually deaf patients.

O. Deguine, MD, Service d'ORL et Otoneurologie, Hôpital Purpan, place du Dr-Baylac, F–31059 Toulouse Cedex (France)

Fraysse B, Deguine O (eds): Cochlear Implants: New Perspectives.
Adv Otorhinolaryngol. Basel, Karger, 1993, vol 48, pp 146–152

Prognostic Factors in 187 Adults Provided with the Nucleus Cochlear Mini-System 22

E. Lehnhardt, A. Aschendorff

Hals-Nasen-Ohrenklinik der Medizinischen Hochschule Hannover, BRD

The predictability of the results of treatment with cochlear implants requires a sufficiently large number of patients and an observation period of several years. We published our first contribution on this subject, based on 4 years' experience, in 1988 [1].

For the statements made for this presentation, we reviewed findings from 187 of 209 adults who had been fitted with the Nucleus device from 1984 until the end of 1991. One hundred and seventy-one patients were bilaterally deaf, and an additional 16 patients were also congenitally deaf. Our intention was to concentrate on the age at onset of deafness, duration of deafness, experience with cochlear implant (CI) and the cause of deafness. We excluded patients with only partial insertion of the electrode lead and the promontory test was not taken into consideration.

For the assessment of patient results, classification into groups has proven valuable to us. The classification is based on understanding without lipreading (LR) and differentiates between patients who: (1) Manage speech tracking without lipreading (group I). (2) Cannot do speech tracking without LR, but understand consonants without lipreading (group II). (3) Can only recognize vowels without lipreading (group III).

The importance of the earliest possible cochlear implant treatment in adults, regarding the expected benefits, can be deduced from a comparison of the duration of the deafness in relation to the patient's age at the time of onset (fig. 1). Individuals deaf from birth, or from earliest childhood – who are now adults – remained exclusively in groups III or II, while group I consisted largely of subjects with deafness of later onset – after the age of 18 years. The shorter the length of deafness, the more apparent was this

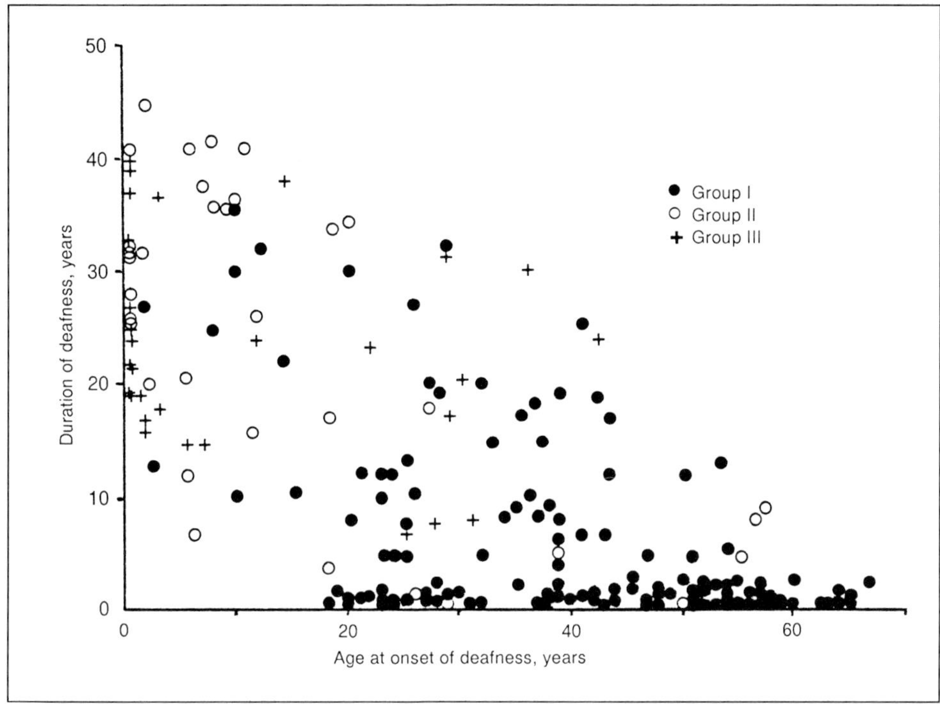

Fig. 1. Comparison of duration of deafness with patient's age at onset of deafness in all the 187 patients fitted with the Nucleus device.

finding. The age at the time of onset of deafness, however, after the age of 18 years is of no significance.

If one limits this relationship to patients with *progressive* hearing loss (n = 52), then the observation that shorter duration of deafness is associated with benefit becomes all the more apparent (fig. 2).

The good benefit obtained in the progressively deaf patients can be explained by the histologic finding of a moderate loss of neurons, in spite of extensive atrophy of the cochlear duct. An additional positive note is that most of the patients in this progressively deaf group had many years experience with hearing aids.

Patients becoming deaf as a result of *meningitis* (n = 44) show a marked influence of age in relation to onset and duration of deafness (fig. 3). That is, the later they became deaf, and the shorter the time they

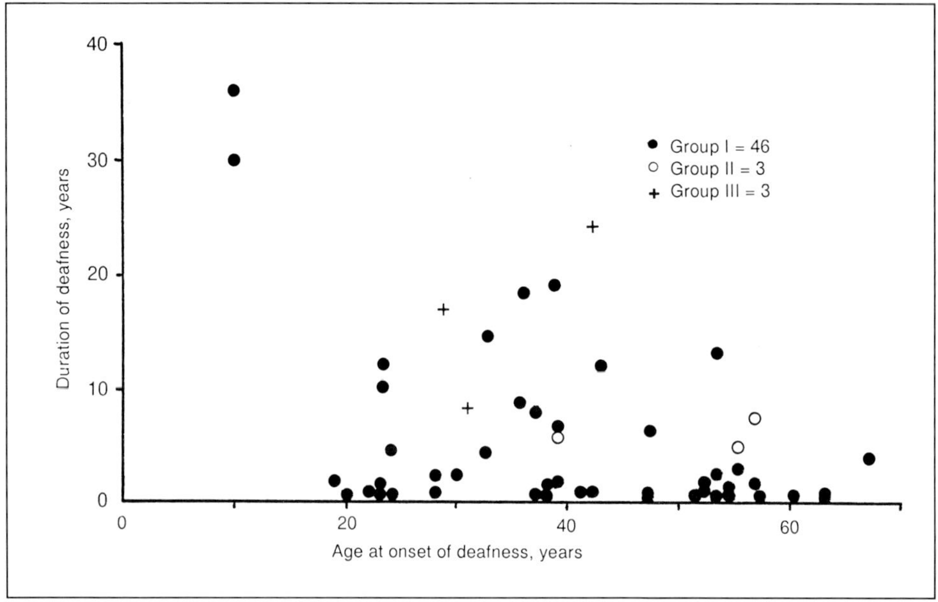

Fig. 2. Same comparison as in figure 1, but in patients with progressive hearing loss only (n = 52).

were deaf, the greater was their chance to make it into group I. Again, there were 5 patients who had been deaf for about 30 years but who, nevertheless, achieved open-set speech understanding.

For those deafened by meningitis, the results considering temporal bone histology proved to be less favorable. Nevertheless, they are better than expected. Following a *bacterial*-meningogenic labyrinthitis, loss of the neuronal structures occurs largely in parallel with fibrotic or bony obliteration of the cochlear spaces. Consequently, selection for cochlear implantation automatically relies upon whether or not there is a sufficiently open lumen for the intracochlear placement of the electrodes. With *complete* obliteration, the neuronal structures are completely missing [2]. Such pictures should give food for thought to those who still believe that they can effectively treat even a white cochlea with an implant. That means at least decades after the onset of deafness the ganglion cell layers are empty or ganglion cells will survive in the obliterated cochlea for a short period after the onset of deafness only.

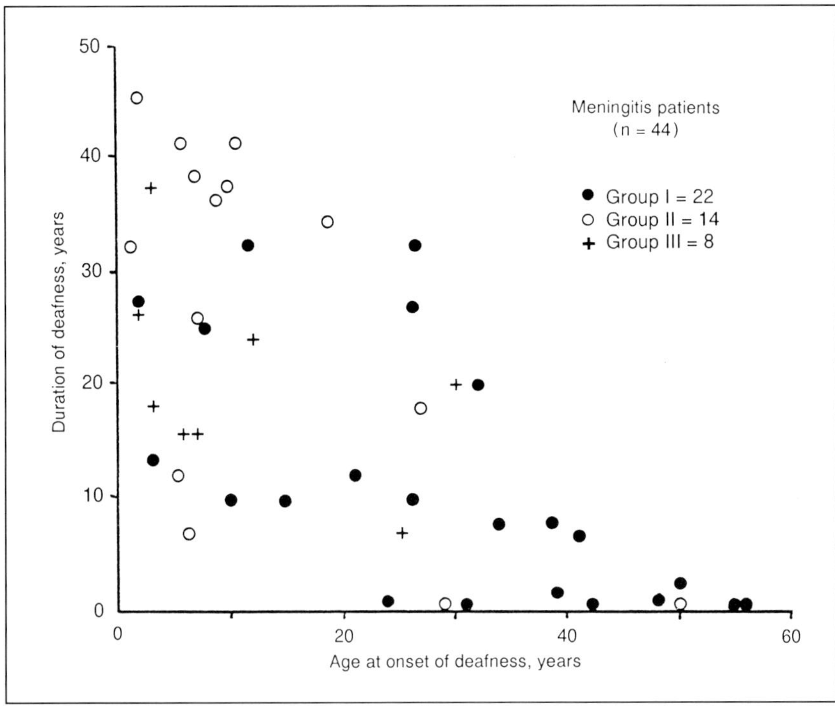

Fig. 3. Influence of age in relation to onset and duration of deafness in 44 patients who became deaf as a result of meningitis.

Relatively favorable results are to be expected with *hematogenic-viral* labyrinthitis – in contrast to meningogenic-bacterial inflammation – which develops primarily in the endolymphatic space. Here, a practically normal neuronal population has still been observed even after many years [3, 4]. On the other hand, the results for *meningogenic*-viral infection, which leads to as much as 2/3 loss of neurons, are different according to the histological findings in 2 patients as reported by Otte et al. [4] (fig. 4).

Concerning the experience with cochlear implants, the rate of understanding for speech tracking clearly does not improve *within-group I.* Clearly, even in speech tracking *with* lipreading (n = 187) there was no longer any marked improvement within this group. Further improvement is in fact almost impossible, because many of these patients – already in group I – already come near to the value of 100 wpm.

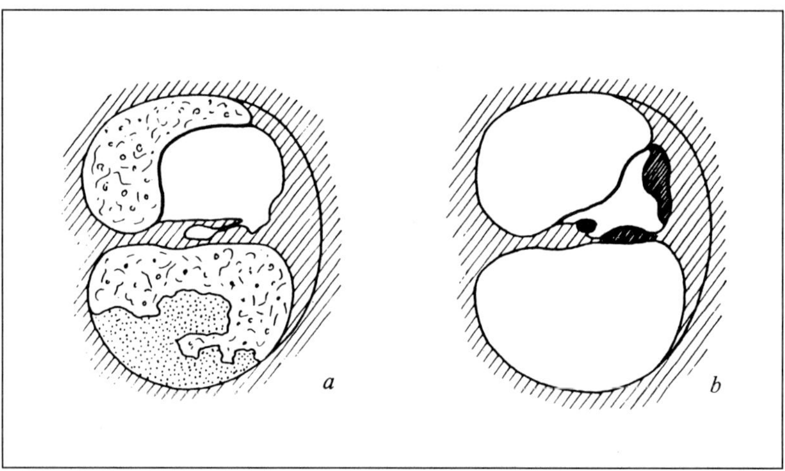

Fig. 4. Scheme of pathology of bacterial (*a*) and viral (*b*) labyrinthitis. From Spoendlin [2], p. 51.

The classification of all of our 187 patients, broken down according to the etiology of deafness and to their inclusion into groups I-III, is shown in table 1. It can be seen that 18 cases are listed under 'other etiologies'. This heterogenous patient population shows about the same distribution into groups I–III as the population of patients who became deaf due to *trauma* (n = 17). The etiology of trauma may include fracture of the temporal bone (n = 11), surgical intervention resulting in immediate deafness (n = 2), and deaf patients without obvious fracture (n = 4). Patients with deafness due to temporal bone *fracture* were, without exception, treated with the cochlear implant very early, and 3 remained in group II in spite of – or because of? – their young age (18–26 years); one remained in group III, probably due to an additional brainstem injury. Of the patients *without* obvious fracture, three made it into group I and one made it into group II. The 2 patients who went deaf following tympanoplasty trauma both made it into group I.

According to the literature, following a fracture, the chance of retention of the integrity of the neuronal structures is slight – especially if the patients are available for cochlear implant treatment only decades after the trauma. After 4 months, neuronal degeneration is still held within reasonable limits, after 30 years it reaches 70%, and after 60 years almost 100%

Table 1. Patient classification

Etiology	n	Group I	Group II	Group III
Progressive hearing loss	52	46	3	3
Meningitis	44	22	14	8
Other etiologies	18	11	6	1
Trauma	17	12	4	1
Congenital	16	–	4	12
Ototox. med.	13	9	4	–
Otosclerosis	8	7	–	1
Acute hearing loss	6	6	–	–
Otitis media	4	2	–	2
Mumps	3	2	–	1
Familial progressive	3	3	–	–
Lues	3	2	–	1
Total	187	122	35	30

Mean age at onset of deafness = 29.9 years (0–67); mean duration of deafness = 12.2 years (0.1–45); mean use of cochlea implant = 3.5 years (0.2–7.5); mean speech tracking = 40.3 wpm (10–92).

[2, 4, 5]. These percentages relate to cranial trauma *with* fracture; *without* fracture, one can hope for a survival rate of the ganglion cells of *more* than 30% [6]. This may well explain why 3 of our 4 patients in this category were in group I.

The findings for the *congenitally* deaf adults were extremely unfavorable. There were none in group I, 4 in group II, and 12 in group III. The indication for cochlear implantation should be extremely strict for the deaf-born population of adults. Even patients who became deaf after meningitis when very young (n = 6) remained in group III.

Of our 13 patients with *ototoxic* deafness, 2 had already become deaf in early childhood. They remained in group II, as did 2 other patients who had become deaf at the ages of 35 and 36 years, respectively. The remaining 9 patients made it into group I – obviously with increasing benefit the longer the experience with the cochlear implant.

The prospects for patients going deaf due to *otosclerosis* can be assessed as positive (n = 8). In otosclerotic patients, the results of the operation are determined by either the otosclerosis which ultimately leads to inner ear deafness with partial obliteration of the scala tympani, or by acute labyrinthitis following surgical intervention at the oval window. Accordingly, the results could be different. Of our 8 otosclerotic patients, none – unfortunately – belonged to the acutely deaf.

Basically, good progress is also shown in the *acutely* deaf (n = 6) and the patients with *familial* deafness (n = 3) who we classify separately from the progressively deaf patients.

The classification of the clinical observations on the one hand, and of the morphological data on the other, will allow more reliable prognostic statements as the patient population becomes larger. Nevertheless, our current knowledge cannot allow us to deny cochlear implant treatment simply because of the only limited prospects of success. Even a partial success can be beneficial to these patients.

One oftern important factor of the unfavorable prognosis will increasingly lose its influence: patients with long-term deafness will more rarely seek cochlear implant treatment (fig. 1). Therefore, for the future, we hope for more uniform – and better – results.

References

1 Lehnhardt E: Cochlear Implant: Prognose-Faktoren. Auris Nasus Larynx 1989; 16(suppl 1):1–8.

2 Spoendlin H: Anatomisch-pathologische Aspekte der Elektrostimulation des ertaubten Innenohres. Arch Otorhinolaryngol 1979;223:1–75.

3 Lindsay JR: Profound childhood deafness inner ear pathology. Ann Otol Rhinol Laryngol 1973;82(suppl):1–121.

4 Otte J, Schuknecht HF, Kerr AG: Ganglion cell populations in normal and pathological human cochleae. Implications for cochlear implantation. Laryngoscope 1978;88:1231.

5 Kerr A, Schuknecht HF: The spiral ganglion in profound deafness. Acta Otolaryngol (Stockh) 1968;(suppl 226):1–76.

6 Lindsay JR, Hinojosa R: The acoustic ganglion in profound sensoneural deafness; in Naunton RF, Fernandes C (eds): Evoked Electrical Activity in the Auditory Nervous System. New York, Academic Press, 1978, p 301.

Professor Dr. Dr. E. Lehnhardt, Siegesstrasse 15, D–30175 Hannover (FRG)

Fraysse B, Deguine O (eds): Cochlear Implants: New Perspectives.
Adv Otorhinolaryngol. Basel, Karger, 1993, vol 48, pp 153–167

Multivariate Predictors of Success with Cochlear Implants[1]

B.J. Gantz[a], *G.G. Woodworth*[b], *J.F. Knutson*[c], *P.J. Abbas*[a], *R.S. Tyler*[a]

[a] Department of Otolaryngology – Head and Neck Surgery;
[b] Department of Statistics and Actuarial Science and Division of Biostatistics, and
[c] Department of Psychology, University of Iowa, Iowa City, Iowa, USA

The cochlear implant has become a reliable and effective method for rehabilitation of profound deafness. The vast majority of postlingually deafened adults and children are able to achieve some sound-only word understanding with multichannel cochlear implant systems [1–3]. Congenital and prelingually deafened children are also demonstrating some remarkable gains with multichannel devices [4]. Event though dramatic results are obtained by some subjects, unfortunately other implant recipients achieve only modest benefits. We have been unable to preoperatively predict the level of performance for an individual. Several factors such as etiology of deafness, IQ, and preoperative promontory stimulation data have not been effective indicators of performance [1–5]. The ability to predict outcome becomes increasingly more important as implant systems improve and we begin to alter implant selection criteria to include subjects with more hearing. Before recommending an implant, the probability of improvement compared to their performance with a hearing aid must be known.

We are presently engaged in a prospective clinical trial of different multichannel cochlear implants. One of the aims of this study is to develop predictors of success with a multichannel cochlear prosthesis. This report will describe our ability to predict audiologic performance based on a multivariate analysis of 48 subjects' preoperative historical audiologic, psycho-

[1] Supported in part by Research Grant DC00242 from the National Institutes of Health/NIDCD and Grant RR59 from the General Clinical Research Centers Program, Division of Research Resources, NIH, and the Iowa Lions Sight and Hearing Foundation.

logic, and electrophysiologic profiles. This information was used to construct percentile and probability curves of audiologic performance at 9 months based on an individual's preoperative predictive index.

Materials and Methods

Subjects

Preoperative and 9-month postoperative data were obtained from 48 consecutively referred postlingual profoundly deaf adults participating in the Iowa Cochlear Implant research project. Criteria for inclusion in this series include: bilateral profound deafness (pure tone average > 90 dB HL), postlingual deafness (lost hearing after learning language and score within norms established for hearing 10 years olds) [6], word understanding with appropriate hearing aid of 4% or less on CID W-22 or NU-6 word lists when presented at 60 dB HL and are 18 years of age or older. Twenty-two females and 26 males ranging in age from 22 to 73 years (mean 52 years, SD 14 years) were implanted with a cochlear prosthesis. The duration of their profound deafness was 1–47 years (mean 13 years, SD 11 years).

Procedure

Candidates meeting the preliminary criteria for receiving a cochlear implant participate in an extensive medical, audiological, electrophysiological, and psychological assessment as previously described [1]. The psychological battery covers a wide variety of attributes from intelligence to cognitive ability and is described in detail by Knutson et al. [7]. The research protocol requires evaluation prior to implantation and at 1, 9, 18, 30, 40, and 54 months postimplantation. To ensure compliance with this schedule, and because many of the test procedures require participants to be able to respond to a broad range of test materials, several psychological factors were included in the final selection criteria, inlcuding lack of psychiatric illness or personality disorder and a measured intelligence above 74 on the Wechsler Adult Intelligence Scale (WAIS).

Subjects electing to participate in the research protocol were prospectively randomized to receive either the Nucleus multichannel implant [8] (n = 24) or the Ineraid (Symbion) multichannel system [9] (n = 24).

The postoperative audiologic assessment was performed uniformly in a sound field at 65 dB SPL. Subjects were allowed to adjust their speech processors to the most comfortable level. Test materials were recorded on audiotape or laser videodisc. Speakers were unfamiliar to the subjects, and only one presentation of an item was allowed. None of the test material was used for rehabilitation. Tests described in this report were administered in a sound-only condition.

The audiologic battery consists of tests from the Minimal Auditory Capabilities Battery (MAC) [9] and tests developed at The University of Iowa [11, 12]. The test battery measures the subjects' ability to recognize environmental sounds, assess word recognition in sentences (Iowa Sentence Test Without Context) and isolation (Nu-6 Monosyllabic Word Test Videodisc). Phoneme recognition was measured with the Iowa Videodisc Medial Consonant Test, Iowa Videodisc Vowel Test, and NU-6 Test. Performance in noise was evaluated with the Spondee 4-Choice in Noise Test.

Table 1. Nine-month audiologic performance (percent values)

	Range	Mean	SD
Iowa Sentence Test Without Context – sound only			
All cases (n = 48)	0–96	34	29
Nucleus (n = 24)*	0–91	38	32
Ineraid (n = 24)*	0–96	30	26
NU-6 Word Understanding – sound only			
All cases (n = 48)	0–46	10	11
Nucleus (n = 24)*	0–36	12	11
Ineraid (n = 24)*	0–46	8	11

* Differences between Nucleus and Ineraid subjects are not significant at $p < 0.05$.

Data Analysis

In this report we investigate the ability to predict audiologic performance after 9 months of implant usage based on preoperative subject profiles. There are several methods of obtaining multivariate analysis. In this paper, detailed methodology is described in order to clarify our techniques for other investigators. The audiologic performance measures are percent correct scores on the Iowa Laser Videodisc Sentence Test, NU-6, Environmental Sounds Test, Consonant Confusion Test, Vowel Confusion Test, and Spondee in Noise Test, all audition only. Presurgical subject profiles were related to postsurgical audiologic scores by means of Pearson Product Moment Correlation Coefficients. Presurgical variables which accounted for 10% or more of the variation in one or more variables of the audiologic battery were identified. Parsimonious subsets of preoperative predictors were selected by applying Mallows Cp Criterion [13]. A predictive index was then developed using multivariate analysis. Smoothed percentile curves were fitted to graphs of outcome versus predictive index.

Results

The audiologic performance of this prospectively randomized group of subjects is similar to other reported series of multichannel cochlear implants in postlingually deafened adults [1, 2]. A wide range of open-set word understanding among subjects is evident (table 1) ranging from 0 to 96% correct on the Iowa Sentence Without Context (mean 34%, SD 29.4%) in the sound-only condition at the 9-month evaluation period. Similar variability is seen in the NU-6 word scores (range 0–46%, mean 10.4%, SD 11.3%). It is of interest to note that there are no significant differences in speech understanding between the Nucleus and Ineraid implant groups even though they employ different electrode configurations and speech coding algorithms.

The Pearson Product Moment correlations between preoperative variables and postoperative audiologic outcome measures administered in the sound-only condition at 9 months are seen in table 2. Correlations accounting for 10% or more of the variance are shown (r > 0.32 or r <

Table 2. Correlations[1] of presurgical measures with 9-month audiology

Predictors	Audiologic measures[2]						
	SNT	CNS	NU6 WRD	NU6 PHN	ENV SND	VWL	SPN
History							
Years profound hearing loss	–48	–40	–45	–49	·	–40	–49
Age at implantation	–34	·	–45	–38	–40	·	·
Etiology	·	·	·	·	·	·	·
Audiology							
Number of frequencies with detectable hearing	37	·	31	·	39	30	·
Pure tone thresholds							
250 Hz	·	·	·	·	–53	·	·
500 Hz	·	·	·	·	·	·	·
1,000 Hz	·	·	·	·	·	·	·
2,000 Hz	·	·	·	·	·	·	·
4,000 Hz	·	·	·	·	·	·	·
8,000 Hz	·	·	·	·	·	·	·
Sentences (visual)	·	34	35	·	·	39	·
Consonants (visual)	38	44	40	39	48	52	·
Electrophysiology (n = 29)							
Round window stimulation (125 Hz)							
Dynamic range	35	·	37	37	·	·	·
Loudness growth slope	·	·	–35	–37	·	·	37
Gap detection	·	·	·	–37	·	·	–45

[1] Correlations accounting for 10% of variance or more are shown (r > 0.32 or r < –0.32). Not all of these are significant due to reduced sample sizes for some variables.
[2] Iowa Laser Videodisc Sentences (SNT) and Consonants (CNS). NU6 Words (WRD) and Phonemes (PHN), Iowa Environmental Sounds Test (ENV SND), Vowel Confusion Test (VWL), Spondee Test (SPN).

Table 2 (continued)

Predictors	Audiologic measures[2]						
	SNT	CNS	NU6 WRD	NU6 PHN	ENV SND	VWL	SPN
Psychological							
CPHI							
Communication performance							
Social importance	36	·	37	41	43	43	36
Home score	·	·	·	·	·	·	·
Home importance	·	·	·	35	35	34	36
Communication environment							
Behavior of others	·	·	·	·	·	·	·
Attitude of others	·	·	·	·	·	·	·
Communication strategies							
Maladaptive behaviors	·	·	·	·	·	·	·
Verbal strategies	·	·	39	40	40	38	·
Nonverbal strategies	44	42	40	47	45	·	·
Personal adjustment							
Acceptance of loss	·	·	·	·	·	·	·
Exaggeration of responsibility	·	·	·	·	·	·	·
WAIS-R (all IQ scales)	·	·	·	·	·	·	·
Ravens matrices (all scales)	·	·	·	·	·	·	·
Benton Visual Retention Test	·	·	·	·	·	·	·
Wechsler Memory Test	·	·	·	·	·	·	·
Multilingual aphasia	·	·	·	·	·	·	·
Beck depression index	·	−32	·	·	·	·	·
MMPI							
Scale K	·	·	·	·	·	·	34
Scale 5	·	·	·	·	·	·	·
Scale 9	·	·	·	·	·	·	·
Scale A	·	·	·	−34	·	−34	·
Scale Mac	·	·	·	·	·	−43	−38
Social anxiety and distress	·	·	·	·	·	·	·
Rathus Assertiveness Scale	·	·	·	·	·	·	·
Health locus of control	·	·	·	·	·	·	·
Krantz Health Opinion Survey							
Total	51	·	46	43	·	35	·
Information seeking	36	·	·	·	·	·	·
Behavioral involvement	53	34	51	47	·	38	34
Cognitive tests							
Probability Learning Task	·	·	·	·	·	·	·
Signal Detection Score	·	·	37	38	38	41	48
Sequence Completion Task	·	43	34	34	·	41	59

Table 3. Proportion of variance[1] of 9-month audiologic battery explained singly by seven presurgical predictors

Predictors	Audiologic measures[2]							
	SNT	CNS	NU6 WRD	NU6 PHN	ENV SND	VWL	SPN	mean[3]
Years of profound deafness (log)	28	22	28	23	7	20	22	21
Iowa Laser Videodisc Consonant Test – vision only	14	19	9	7	23	28	20	17
CPHI Non-Verbal Communication Strategies Scale	25	17	17	13	19	12	11	16
Knutson's Signal Detection Score	7	9	13	15	15	17	23	14
Krantz Health Opinion Survey total	19	6	17	12	3	11	6	11
Number of frequencies with detectable hearing	14	7	10	7	15	9	4	9
Dynamic range of 125 Hz (round window)	7	6	9	8	0	3	6	6

[1] Proportion of variance explained by each predictor used alone.
[2] See table 2 for variable identifications.
[3] Mean proportion of variance explained.

–0.32). Additional variables of interest such as etiology of deafness and IQ are presented to demonstrate their negligible correlations with outcome measures. A set of the most significant predictor variables was identified from this table by selecting those measures which seemed to have the most consistently high correlations over the entire auditory battery, and were not redundant with other variables. Mallow's Cp criterion was then used to select an efficient subset of predictor variables [13]. Cp selects predictors by balancing the ability to predict the 48 current cases (multiple R^2) against the potential for reduced predictive power in future cases due to chance selection of useless predictors.

Cp is not related to significance levels in any simple way and we do not report them here. The set of predictor variables selected by Cp is only one of several roughly equally useful sets of variables; thus exclusion of a variable does not imply that it has no predictive power.

Table 3 lists the chosen predictor variables and the mean proportion of variance in the audiologic outcome measures explained by each predictor. Clearly the round window preoperative measure was at best of marginal importance in our experience. Further analysis (table 4) indicates

Table 4. Proportion of variance[1] of 9- and 18-month audiologic battery explained jointly by seven presurgical predictors

Predictors	Audiologic measures[2]						
	SNT	CNS	NU6 WRD	NU6 PHN	ENV SND	VWL	SPN
Years of profound deafness (log)	28	22	28	22	4	16	19
Iowa Laser Videodisc Consonant Test – vision only	1	16	–	–	23	28	5
CPHI Non-Verbal Communication Strategies Scale	21	8	14	11	12	3	9
Knutson's Signal Detection Score	4	3	11	12	8	4	23
Krantz Health Opinion Survey total	12	–	7	4	–	1	–
Number of frequencies with detectable hearing	2	1	1	–	2	6	–
Dynamic range at 125 Hz (round window)	–	–	–	1	2	–	1
Total[3]	67	50	62	50	51	58	56

[1] Proportion of variance explained in the order of entry of variables under forward selection. All variables predicting above chance are shown.
[2] See table 2 for variable identifications.
[3] Proportion of variance (R-squared) explained jointly by the predictors.

that between 67 and 50% of the total variation in each of the variables in the audiologic battery is predictable. Inspection of tables 3 and 4 indicates that the most useful single predictor is duration of profound deafness expressed as the logarithm (i.e. the harm produced by one additional year of deafness declines with number of years of deafness). The second most useful is speech reading ability demonstrated on the vision-only Iowa Consonant Confusion Test, although this variable ultimately proved to provide little additional predictive power beyond that provided by the psychological variables. In addition, the communication profile for the hearing impaired (CPHI) Non-Verbal Communication Strategy, Krantz Health Opinion Survey Total (HOS), Cognitive Signal Detection Score and a (0/1) variable indicating greater than four frequencies of measureable hearing all proved useful in combination. It should be noted in the joint analysis that the round window measure had no useful predictive power beyond that provided by other, noninvasive measures.

Six of the preoperative predictors were reduced to a single predictive index by linear regression of the predictors on the optimal monotone transformation of the auditional only sentence and NU-6 scores at nine months as determined by SAS PROC TRANSREG [14]. The predictive index is a weighted sum of the predictor variables as seen below:

Predictive index =	−7.9	
	−13.9	log duration of deafness
	+04.2	Cognitive Signal Detection Score
	+02.3	HOS Total Score
	+12.2	CPHI Non-Verbal Communication Strategy Score
	+15.4	hearing present at more than 4 frequencies
	+0.36	Vision-Only Consonant Test Score

Mean values of the predictor variables were substituted for missing data. The predictive index was developed by nonlinear canonical correlation analysis using SAS procedure TRANSREG [14]. Because of the adaptive nature of that procedure, reliable significance levels cannot be attributed to individual predictors; however, in stepwise linear regressions for each of the seven dependent variables in the audiologic battery, duration of deafness was significant at the 0.01 level for every variable except the environmental sounds test and each of the other predictors was a significant predictor at the 0.01 level for at least 1 of the 7 audiologic outcome measures.

Ranges of the predictor variables were:

Predictor	Mean	Range
log duration of deafness	2.1	0–3.9
Cognitive Signal Detection Score	0	−4.4–1.6
HOS Total Score	5.6	0–15.0
CPHI Non-Verbal Communication Strategy Score	4.0	21.0–5.0
Hearing present at more than 4 frequencies		0/1
Vision-Only Consonant Test Score	28.6	16–49

Thus, the predictive index could be as small as −49, for a subject with the least favorable combination of predictors, and as large as 127, for a subject with the most favorable. None of our subjects was either extreme – the predictive index ranged from −15.3 to 94.1 with mean 34.8 and SD 25.2.

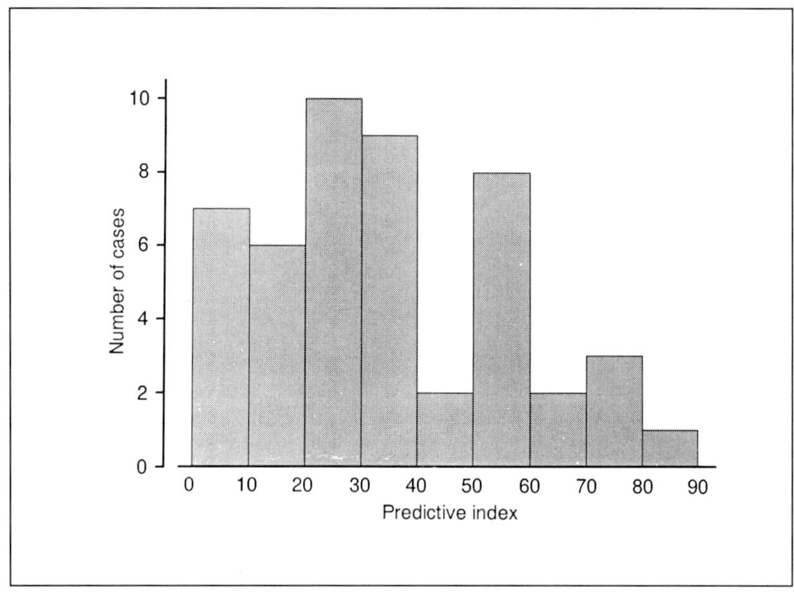

Fig. 1. Distribution of the predictive index for 48 subjects. Negative values have been replaced by zero.

The distribution of predictive index scores across our subject population is shown in figure 1.

Figures 2 and 3 display individual audiologic performance scores at 9 months for the sentence and NU-6 word tests and demonstrate the ability of the predictive index to forecast the level of audiologic performance. Plotted on the graphs are the median and the 10th, 25th, 75th, and 90th percentiles of actual performance at each predictive score. These curves were obtained with a multistage smoothing process using the TRANSREG procedure in the Statistical Analysis System, Release 6 [14] (the smoothing process consisted of detrending the data with a 3-knot monotone quadratic spline, computing moving percentiles using a 20-case window, restoring the trend, and smoothing the re-trented moving percentile curves with 2- or 3-knot monotone quadratic splines). Figure 2 illustrates that for subjects with a preoperative predictive index of 20, the median predicted performance on the Iowa Sentence Test in the sound-only condition at 9 months is about 12% correct. Conversely, for subjects with a

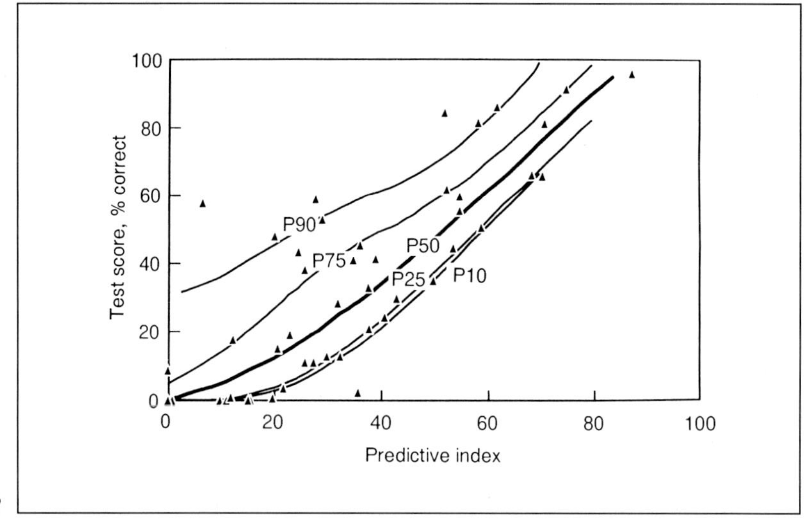

2

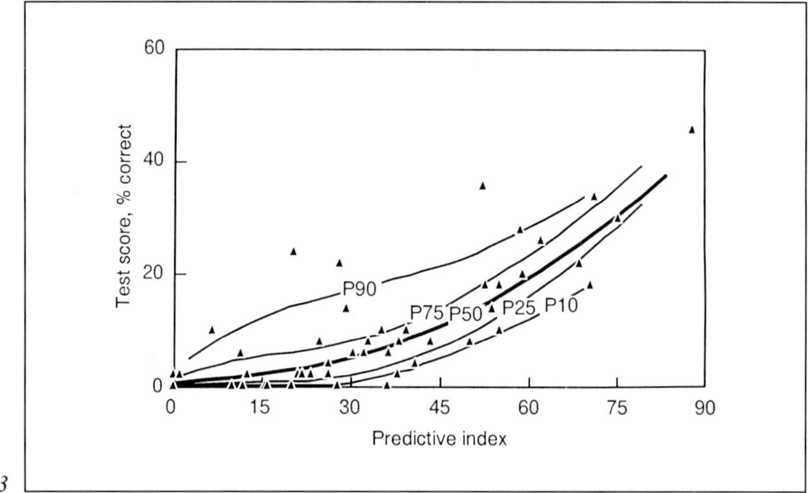

3

Fig. 2. Audition-only sentence scores for 48 subjects tested approximately nine months after connection of the cochlear implant. Raw data and smoothed percentile curves are plotted against the predictive index. Raw data and smoothed percentile curves are plotted against the predictive index. Smoothed percentiles were obtained by fitting monotone splines to moving percentiles using a 20-case window.

Fig. 3. NU6 word scores for 48 subjects tested approximately nine months after connection of the cochlear implant. Raw data and smoothed percentile curves are plotted against the predictive index. Smoothed percentiles were obtained by fitting monotone splines to moving percentiles using a 20-case window.

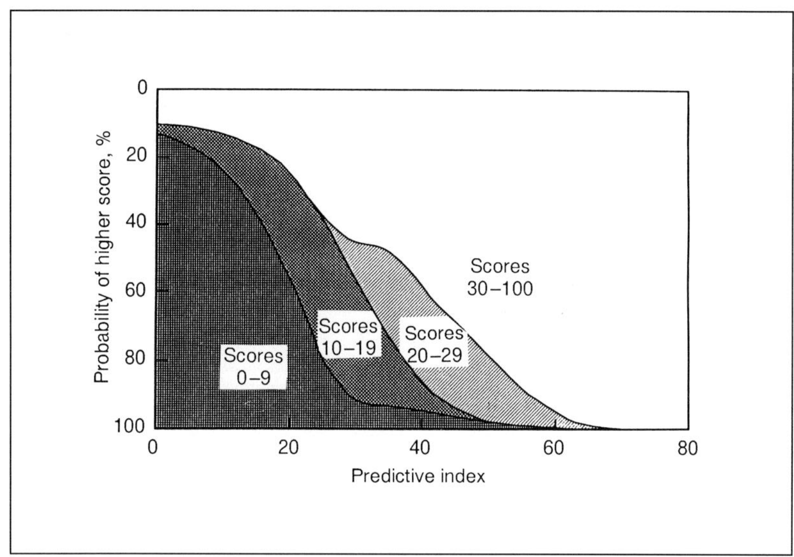

Fig. 4. Estimated probability of exceeding a given score on the Iowa Laser Videodisc Sentence Test administered under audition-only conditions approximately nine months after connection of the cochlear implant. Probabilities of equalling or exceeding 10, 20 and 30% word understanding are plotted as functions of the predictive index. Probability curves were obtained by fitting monotone splines to moving success rates using a 20-case window applied to the data of figure 2, with success defined as a score of 10% or better, 20% or better or 30% or better, respectively.

predictive index of 60 the median performance is 50% at 9 months. Figure 3 provides similar information for NU-6 word understanding in the sound-only condition.

The graphs of test scores versus predictive index were also used to construct probability curves. These curves were made by computing moving frequencies using a 20-case window and smoothing the frequency curves with 2-knot monotone quadratic splines. Figure 4 shows the resulting estimates of the probability of achieving a given word understanding score on the sentence test at nine months based on an individual's predictive index. For example, an individual with a predictive index of 30 has approximately a 90% chance of reaching a 20% or greater score. A subject with a predictive index of 40 has a 95% chance of scoring better than 10%, 85% chance of scoring better than 20%, and a 60% chance of understand-

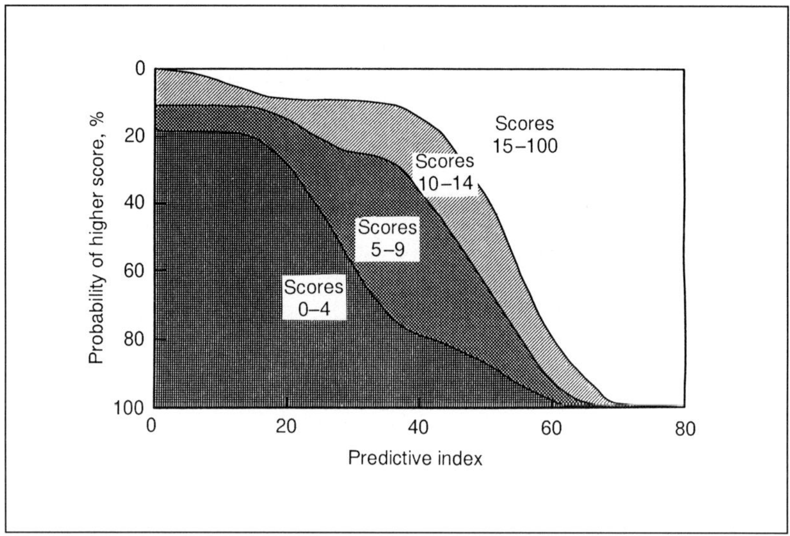

Fig. 5. Estimated probability of exceeding a given word score on the NU6 test administered approximately nine months after connection of the cochlear implant. Probabilities of equaling or exceeding 5, 10 and 15% word understanding are plotted as functions of the predictive index. Probability curves were obtained by fitting monotone splines to moving success rates using a 20-case window applied to the data of figure 3, with success defined as a score of 5% or better, 10% or better or 15% or better, respectively.

ing more than 30% of the words in sentences. The probability of achieving various levels of NU-6 word understanding at 9 months is seen in figure 5.

Discussion

One of the most frequently asked questions which is of great concern to the prospective cochlear implant candidate is what level of audiologic performance cover can be expected with an implant. It is clear that the levels of audiologic performance with multichannel implants cover a broad range. The present study population confirms the variability reported in other studies [1, 2]. Predicting outcome has become one of the most prominent challenges confronting cochlear implant research. Individual characteristics such as etiology of deafness and measured intelligence continue to be disappointing indicators of audiologic outcome. The lack of correlation is evident in table 2 as etiology and WAIS-R scores failed to demonstrate any correlation. It has been necessary to perform more sophisticated analyses combining multichannel measures to arrive at a clearer understanding of performance with an implant. It is encouraging that a predictive index derived from a multiple regression analysis of a weighted linear combination of preoperative measures was able to discriminate among more and less successful implant users.

It is not surprising that duration of profound deafness is a powerful predictor of performance since it may be highly correlated with residual auditory nerve viability. Similarly, hearing at a greater number of frequencies contributes to the predictive index and also reflects some measure of neural integrity. The present population has a high percentage of subjects with no measurable hearing, or hearing at one or two frequencies. As subjects with more hearing are implanted this variable may become a greater distinguishing characteristic of audiologic outcome. The poor predictive performance of the preoperative electrophysiologic measures recorded from round window stimulation including EABR threshold and input/output function was disappointing. It was expected that preoperative round window stimulation would yield useful nerve survival information. The inconsistent responses among the first 29 accrued subjects has led us to discontinue the invasive preoperative round window stimulation for routine candidates. Round window stimulation is still performed on subjects with severe labyrinthitis ossificans, history of trauma, or retrocochlear surgical procedures.

Another important facet of this analysis has been the ability to identify certain psychological variables that impact on audiologic performance. The ability to extract information from sequentially arrayed signals and rapidly process that information as measured by the cognitive signal detection score appears to be relevant to word understanding with an implant. We believe it is likely that the same attentional and cognitive abilities contribute to performance on the preoperative vision-only consonant confusion test and explains why it is a predictor of audiologic outcome. The utility of two self-report measures, the Health Opinion Survey and the nonverbal communication strategy subscale of CPHI, suggests that the level of engagement and participation of a candidate and their efforts to use communication skills also contribute to the overall outcome of cochlear implants.

Jointly, six of the most significant preoperative measures account for 67% of the between-subject variance displayed in the sound-only sentence understanding scores following 9 months of multichannel cochlear implant experience. This predictive index was highly correlated with both the sound-only sentence scores (correlation coefficients = 0.81) and the sound-only NU-6 word understanding (correlation coefficient = 0.78). The probability curves generated by these data will be useful in forecasting the probability of achieving sentence and word understanding with a multichannel cochlear implant based on noninvasive preoperative measures. This information will be helpful in informing postlingually deafened adult cochlear implant candidates about the range of otucomes they are likely to achieve with the present generation of multichannel cochlear implant systems. It is also of interest to note that the type of multichannel implant system does not significantly alter audiologic outcome at 9 months in this prospectively randomized trial. Finally, these methods of data analysis and their results should be useful in guiding future alterations in candidate selection criteria as subjects with more hearing are considered.

References

1 Gantz BJ, Tyler RS, Knutson JF, Woodworth G, Abbas P, McCabe BF, Hinrichs J, Tye-Murray N, Lansing C, Kuk F, Brown C: Evaluation of five different cochlear implant designs: Audiologic assessment and predictors of performance. Laryngoscope 1988;98:1100–1106.

2 Cohen NL, Waltzman SB, Fisher SG: A prospective randomized clinical trial of advanced cochlear implants: Preliminary results of a VA cooperative study. Ann Otol Rhinol Laryngol 1991;100:823–829.

3 Staller SJ, Beiter AL, Brimacombe JA, Mecklenburg DS, Arndt PA: Pediatric performance with the Nucleus 22-channel cochlear implant system. Am J Otol 1991; 12(suppl):126–136.

4 Fryauf-Bertschy H, Tyler R, Kelsay D, Gantz B: Performance over time of congenitally and postlingually deafened children using multichannel cochlear implants. JSHR 1992;35:913–920.

5 Abbas P, Brown C: In Cooper HW (ed): Assessment of Status of the Auditory Nerve in Cochlear Implants: A Practical Guide. London, Whurr, 1991.

6 Quigley SP, Steenkamp M, Power D, Jones B: Test of Syntactive Abilities. Beaverton, Donall, 1978.

7 Knutson JF, Hinrichs JV, Tyler RS, Gantz BJ, Schartz HA, Woodworth G: Psychological predictors of audiological outcomes of multichannel cochlear implants. Ann Otol Rhinol Laryngol 1991;100:817–822.

8 Clark GM, et al: The University of Melbourne-Nucleus Multi-Electrode Cochlear Implant; in Pfaltz CR (ed): Adv Otorhinolar. Basel, Karger, 1987, vol 38.

9 Eddington DK, et al: Auditory prosthesis research with multiple-channel intra-cochlear stimulation in man. Ann Otol Rhinol Laryngol 1978;87(suppl 53):5–39.
10 Owens E, Kessler D, Telleen C, et al: The Minimal Auditory Capabilities Battery. St Louis, Auditec, 1981.
11 Tyler R, Preece J, Lowder M: The Iowa Cochlear Implant Tests. Iowa City, University of Iowa Department of Otolaryngology – Head & Neck Surgery, 1983.
12 Tyler RS, Preece J, Tye-Murray N: The Iowa Phoneme and Sentence Laser Videodisc. Iowa City, University of Iowa Department of Otolaryngology – Head and Neck Surgery, 1986.
13 Weisburg S: Applied Linear Regression, ed 2. New York, Wiley, 1985.
14 SAS Institute Inc, SAS/STAT: User's Guide, version 6, ed 4, vol 2. Cary, SAS Institute Inc, 1990.

Bruce J. Gantz, MD, Department of Otolaryngology – Head and Neck Surgery,
University of Iowa Hospitals and Clinics, Iowa City, IA 52242 (USA)

Fraysse B, Deguine O (eds): Cochlear Implants: New Perspectives.
Adv Otorhinolaryngol. Basel, Karger, 1993, vol 48, pp 168–173

Tinnitus Suppression in Cochlear Implant Users[1]

René Dauman[a], *Richard S. Tyler*[b]

[a] Department of Audiology, CHU Bordeaux and INSERM U.229, Bordeaux, France;
[b] Department of Otolaryngology, Speech Pathology and Audiology, University of Iowa, Iowa City, Iowa, USA

Postlingually deaf adults may be severely affected by tinnitus. When the suitability of a cochlear implant is discussed, patients often wish to know if their tinnitus will change after surgery.

Over the past years, several studies have reported tinnitus relief in cochlear implant patients [1]. These studies were generally performed with a single-channel implant. With the 3M-House implant, Berliner et al. [2] observed a tinnitus improvement in 53% of users. With the implant developed in London, Hazell et al. [3] reported a tinnitus improvement in 54% of users. With some of the best single and multichannel implant users, Tyler and Kelsay [4] observed a tinnitus reduction in 81%. A recent study by Gibson [5] on patients with a multichannel implant claimed a reduction of tinnitus in 61% when the device was used for speech perception and 26% when the device was turned on.

Materials and Methods

This preliminary report is limited to 2 postlingually deaf adults implanted with the Nucleus device [6] and complaining of tinnitus. Their tinnitus annoyance was estimated at 22 and 43% in patients 1 and 2, respectively, on the Tinnitus Handicap Questionnaire [7].

[1] This work was supported by the French Ministère de la Recherche et de la Technologie, and the American Tinnitus Association.

We varied the current level, and investigated its relationship to (1) the loudness of stimulus, and (2) the loudness of the tinnitus. The speech processor, a MSP processor (Mini System 22) for patient 1 and a WSP III processor (an older version of the former) for patients 2, was controlled by the Nucleus DPI interface (version 6.53). For a given experiment, we first determined the threshold and the uncomfortable loudness level. Different current levels were selected within the range between threshold and uncomfortable loudness level. They were presented randomly to the patient, typically with 3 replications per current level. For each presentation, the subject was asked to rate on a 0 to 100 scale the loudness of the stimulus (i.e. the sound heard when the electrode was stimulated) and the loudness of his tinnitus.

Results

Figure 1 shows the relationship between the current levels and the loudness ratings of stimulus and tinnitus, using a bipolar stimulation of electrode 15 with a repetition rate of 250 Hz in patient 2 (subject L). The individual data points are given and the line goes through the average values. Two functions are thus obtained: the stimulus loudness growth (dotted line) and the tinnitus reduction curve (solid line). We can define the crossover point as the place where the two functions cross, here at 0.65 mA. Results are presented according to 4 parameters: electrode location, frequency of stimulation, interelectrode distance, and post-stimulus effect.

Electrode Location

In patient 1 (subject F), we first assessed the effect of electrode location, using a bipolar + 1 stimulation mode and a pulse rate of 250 Hz. The crossover point was lower with electrode 12 (0.55 mA) than with electrode 4 (0.7 mA), indicating that less current was needed with the former electrode to reduce tinnitus. Patient 1 reported two annoying tinnitus sounds, a cricket noise (high-pitched) and an ocean noise (lower pitched). He found basal electrode 4 more effective for the cricket and apical electrode 20 better for the ocean. We asked him to indicate the stimulus loudness which he preferred for tinnitus reduction: with both electrodes, the best stimulus loudness was between 20 and 30%, therefore the best current level was around 0.55 mA.

In patient 2, only electrodes 21 to 11 were available due to a severe labyrinthine fracture. We assessed the effect of electrode location with a bipolar stimulation (which he used for 2 years) and a 250 Hz pulse rate.

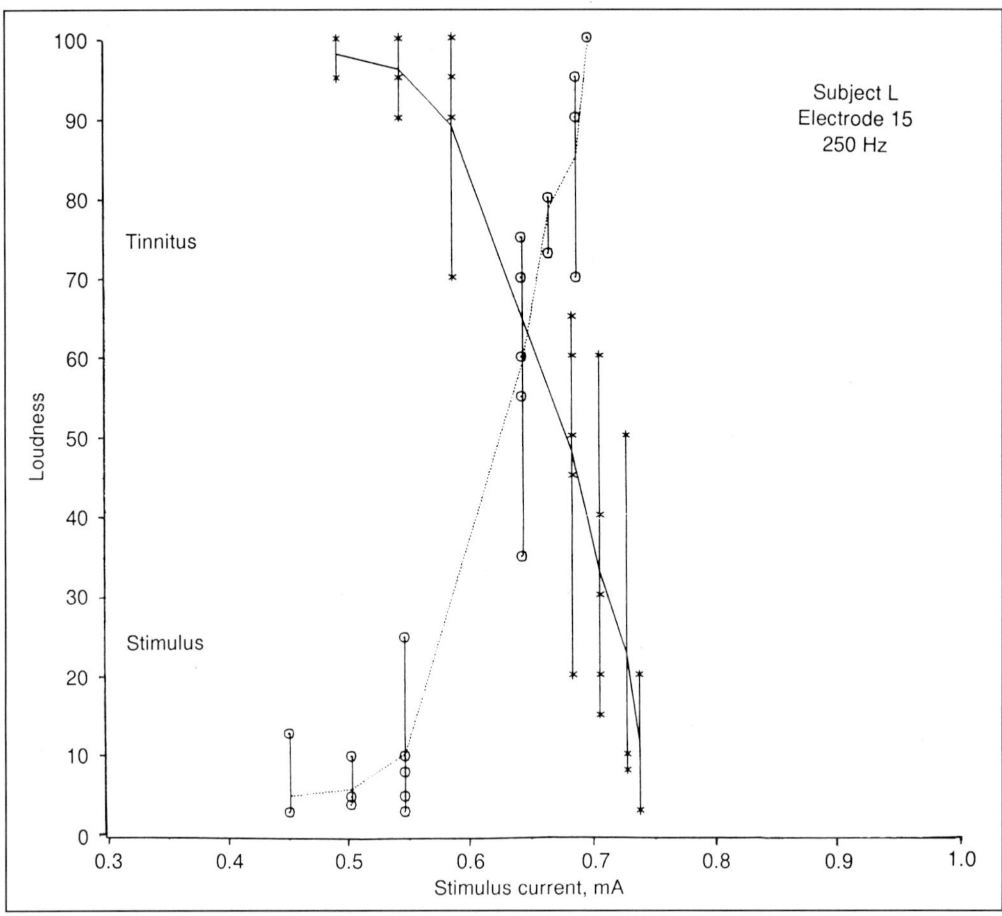

Fig. 1. The loudness of stimulus and of tinnitus is shown on the vertical axis on a 0–100 scale as a function of the current level expressed in mA. The dotted line in the figure shows the loudness of the stimulus, the solid line shows the loudness of the tinnitus. The crossover point, where the stimulus and the tinnitus have about the same loudness, is located around 0.65 mA. Results for subject L.

With electrodes 21 and 11 the crossover point was around 0.8 mA, therefore it required high current levels to suppress tinnitus. With stimulation of electrode 13, a very low level of current was needed to suppress tinnitus (crossover point around 0.4 mA), whereas with electrode 15 the preferred current level was around 0.65 mA.

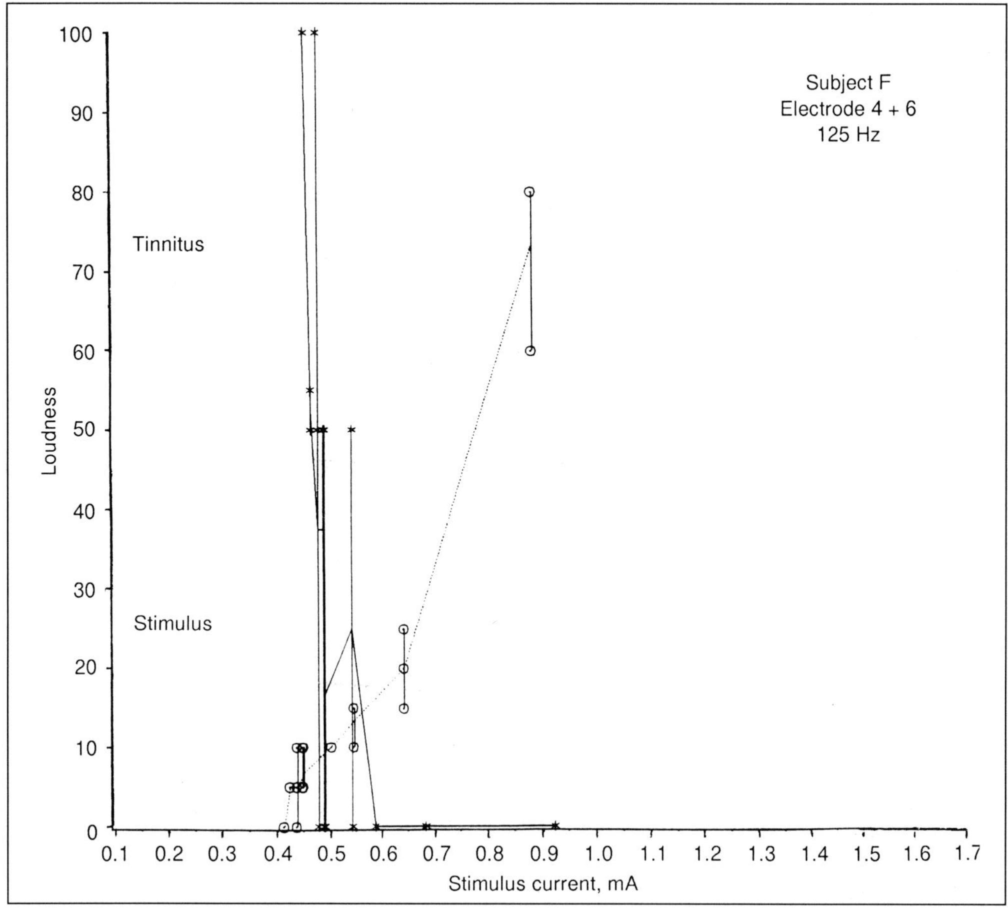

Fig. 2. Stimulus (dotted line) and tinnitus (solid line) loudness as a function of current level for subject F. Tinnitus suppression is obtained at low current levels and a low stimulus loudness of 15%.

Frequency of Stimulation

In patient 1, we examined the effect of changing the frequency of stimulation on tinnitus suppression, using electrode 4 and a bipolar + 1 stimulation (fig. 2). With a pulse rate of 125 Hz, the reliability of tinnitus ratings was not very good at very low current levels for this patient, but tinnitus suppression was obtained with low stimulus loudness: at 20% of the stimulus loudness the tinnitus was completely suppressed. The crossover point was lower at 125 than 250 Hz. We also tried lower and higher frequencies (80 and 500 Hz), but the patient did not report any additional benefit.

In patient 2 we tested the same 4 frequencies, but with another electrode, apical electrode 21. As in patient 1, a pulse rate of 125 Hz required less current to suppress tinnitus than the frequencies of 80, 250 or 500 Hz.

Interelectrode Distance

Our third area of interest was the effect of the interelectrode distance. In subject 1 the bipolar + 3 stimulation (electrode 4–8) had a crossover point of 0.4 mA, and the bipolar + 1 stimulation (electrode 4–6) had a crossover point of 0.7 mA. In general, the greater the interelectrode distance, the less current was required to suppress tinnitus, at least for the electrodes we tested.

In patient 2, similarly, the bipolar + 3 stimulation (electrode 18–22) took less current to suppress tinnitus than the bipolar + 1 stimulation (electrode 20–22).

Poststimulus Effects

Finally, we were interested in studying these effects during and after a prolonged electrical stimulation. Before stimulation the tinnitus loudness was 100% and the stimulus loudness was obviously 0%. We presented the stimulus at 125 Hz on electrode 21 to patient 2, at the preferred loudness level of 50%, for a duration of 300 s. The stimulus was rated at 60% loudness, and the tinnitus was reduced to around 40% during the stimulation. After stimulation, tinnitus loudness was reduced even lower (to 30%) for a few minutes, and then it returned progressively to 100% after 15 min.

Discussion

Preliminary results show that the electrode position in the cochlea influences the current level required to suppress tinnitus in cochlear implant patients. For instance in patient 2, the stimulation of the extreme electrodes 21 and 11 needed much more current to suppress tinnitus than the stimulation of electrode 13 or, to a lesser extent, 15. This suggests that the effectiveness of current in suppressing tinnitus appears related to a particular electrode location. The findings in patient 1 also indicate that the stimulation of a deeply inserted electrode may be needed in some patients rather than the stimulation of a short insertion. Regarding the pulse rate, if we consider the criteria that the lowest current level is the best for the patient, the frequency of 125 Hz appeared substantially better for tinnitus suppression than 250 or 80 Hz for the 2 subjects examined. In general, the greater the interelectrode distance, the less current was needed to suppress tinnitus. We hope to provide cochlear implant patients with a stimulating program that they could select in a quiet environment or when their tinnitus is especially bothersome.

References

1 Tyler RS, Aran JM, Dauman R: Recent advances in tinnitus. Am J Audiol 1992;1: 36–44.

2 Berliner KI, Cunningham JK, House WF: Effect of the cochlear implant on tinnitus in profoundly deaf patients; in Feldmann H (ed): Proceedings of the III International Tinnitus Seminar, Münster. Karlsruhe, Harsch Verlag, 1987, pp 415–453.

3 Hazell JWP, Meerton LJ, Conway JJ: Electrical tinnitus suppression (ETS) with a single channel cochlear implant. J Laryngol Otol 1989;18:39–44.

4 Tyler RS, Kelsay D: Advantages and disadvantages perceived by some of the better cochlear-implant patients. Am J Otol 1990;11:282–289.

5 Gibson WPR: The effect of electrical stimulation and cochlear implantation on tinnitus; in Aran JM, Dauman R (eds): Proceedings of the IV International Tinnitus Seminar, Bordeaux. Amsterdam, Kugler & Ghedini 1992, pp 403–408.

6 Tong YC, Clark GM, Seligman PM, Patrick JF: Speech-processing for a multiple-electrode cochlear implant hearing prothesis. J Acoust Soc Am 1980;68:1897–1899.

7 Kuk FK, Tyler RS, Russell D, Jordan H: The psychometric properties of a tinnitus handicap questionnaire. Ear Hear 1990;11:434–442.

René Dauman, MD, Department of Audiology, Hôpital Pellegrin,
F–33076 Bordeaux Cedex (France)

Fraysse B, Deguine O (eds): Cochlear Implants: New Perspectives.
Adv Otorhinolaryngol. Basel, Karger, 1993, vol 48, pp 174–176

Sound Localization with the Ineraid Cochlear Implant

Roger F. Gray, David M. Baguley

Department of Audiology, Addenbrooke's Hospital, Cambridge, UK

Patients with the Ineraid cochlear implant have been demonstrated to have a wide range of auditory abilities, including environmental sound perception, improvement of communication with lipreading, and for some patients the ability to perceive well with hearing alone. With this in mind we wished to determine the ability of our patients to localize the source of a sound in space, as this ability has uses in social interaction, in road safety, and in workplace safety, and so would be of great benefit to cochlear implant users. Furthermore, we considered that the compressed analogue (CA) stimulation strategy employed by the Ineraid does not manipulate the sound signal in such a manner that localization information might be lost, which may be the case in devices using a feature extraction algorithm.

It must be borne in mind that the cochlear implant user has still a unilateral dead ear, and so if any sound localization is achieved it will be analogous to monaural localization in hearing subjects. This monaural condition does not allow the subject to make use of time and phase differences in the stimulus unless head movements are allowed, and it has been noted that if this is the case monaural localization can be as accurate as binaural [1], and that this ability may be related to the pinna transforming sound as it enters the canal. Moore [2] notes, however, that this lack of superior ability in the binaural condition may be a function of the lack of sensitivity of the test rather than an equality of ability in the binaural and monaural conditions.

This study therefore undertook to investigate the sound localization ability of our patients in two ways: to ask the patients to rate their own ability; and then to test a small number of patients to determine if they were accurate.

Method

Self-Rating

Patients were asked to give a value to their ability to find the source of a sound in space against an arbitrary 'normal' value of 100%. They were also asked if this localization was easier on the side of their implant.

Testing

Patients were asked to point to the source of a sound in the plane of their implant microphone. The stimuli used were a 1,000-Hz warble tone, and a 1,000-Hz centred narrow band noise for 2 s, with a wide-band noise from another speaker masking the sound source movement between trials. The stimuli were presented in a sound proofed room at 40 dBSL, thresholds being determined perpendicular to the patients ear. This maximised the amount of intensity information available, as the stimuli would therefore be quieter when presented to the other ear. Ten trials for each patients were presented at positions determined by the calculation of random numbers in the 360° around the patient. Head movements were allowed.

Results

The self-rating of localization ability by the 9 subjects who replied (of 10 contacted) was recorded. The range was between 0 and 70% (mean 25%, SD 25.86). No correlation could be found between discrimination ability (sentences, auditory only) and self-rated localization ability. All patients who felt they had some localization ability (8 of 9 replies) stated that this was easier on the implanted side.

On testing 3 patients with our protocol it became apparent that this procedure was not sensitive enough to demonstrate the ability that our patients felt they had (self-rated ability was 70, 65 and 10%). All three made large errors (± 87° on average) and no difference was evident between patients and between the tone and noise stimuli. It was interesting to note, however, that in 43% of the trials the subject correctly identified which quadrant the sound source was in. Errors confusing sounds presented from behind with those presented from in front were more common than those confusing side of presentation, though the sample was so small as not to be statistically analyzed. The performance of patients was so poor that a new test protocol is being formulated in the hope that it will be more sensitive to the abilities claimed by the patients.

Discussion

The Cambridge series of patients felt that they had some localization ability. This may consist of the limited ability to identify a quadrant of source, but if so will be useful when the subject can then see the sound source. This ability may be due to the CA strategy employed by the Ineraid device, though a study on patients with the Nucleus device would be of interest. The influence of microphone placement should be considered as if it is the pinnae that allow monaural localization, then the contribution of the pinna will only be evident if an ear canal microphone is empoyed. At present the Ineraid device has a microphone which sits in front of the pinna whereas with the Nucleus device the microphone is placed above the pinna as for a behind the ear hearing aid. Microphone placement should be considered in future cochlear implant designs.

References

1 Freedman SJ, Fisher HG: The role of the pinna in auditory localization; in Freedman SJ (ed): Neuropsychology of Spatially Oriented Behaviour. Chicago, Dorsey Press, 1968.

2 Moore BCJ: An Introduction to the Psychology of Hearing. London, Academic Press, 1982.

Dr. Roger F. Gray, Department of Audiology, Addenbrooke's Hospital, Cambridge CB2 2QQ (UK)

Fraysse B, Deguine O (eds): Cochlear Implants: New Perspectives.
Adv Otorhinolaryngol. Basel, Karger, 1993, vol 48, pp 177–181

Cochlear Implantation in the Deaf Blind

Richard T. Ramsden, Paul Boyd, Ellen Giles, Yvonne Aplin, Vijay Das

Department of Otolaryngology and Centre for Audiology,
University of Manchester, UK

The cochlear implant programme in Manchester commenced in June 1988, since when 34 adults and 2 postlingually deaf children have received multichannel intracochlear devices (35 Nucleus, 1 Ineraid). During this time experience has been gained of the unique problems of the deaf blind, 5 of whom have been implanted.

Patients

During the past 4 years, approximately 200 potential implant recipients have been assessed on the Manchester Royal Infirmary/University of Manchester Cochlear Implant Programme. Thirty-four postlingually deaf adults and 2 postlingually deaf children have received implants, and at present one new implant operation is performed per month. During this time 14 deaf blind patients have been referred for assessment for cochlear implantation. The age range was 19–81 years (mean 48 years). There were 9 males and 5 females. The duration of deafness was 3–59 years (mean 14 years). The duration of blindness was 3–74 years (mean 35 years). Five received implants. Four were implanted in our unit with multichannel devices (Nucleus). One was referred to the UCH unit in London, for a single-channel device after assessment in Manchester. The times since switch on are 38, 30, 18 and 2 months for the multichannel patients and 12 months for the UCH patient. Two patients are awaiting implantation, 2 are in the process of evaluation, and 5 have been turned down for implantation.

Aetiology

Tables 1 and 2 list the causes of the deafness and blindness. One patient had two causes contributing to his deafness. He suffered from Behcet's syndrome and otosclerosis, and lost the hearing in one ear following an unsuccessful stapedectomy. In 6 cases there was a common aetiology for both deafness and blindness (meningitis 2; Usher's syndrome 2; Still's disease 1; Behçet's syndrome).

Table 1. Aetiology of deafness

Meningitis	4
Usher's syndrome	2
Still's disease	1
Congenital	1
Behçet's disease	1
Stapedectomy	1
Myelodysplasia	1
Idiopathic progressive	2
Idiopathic sudden	2

Table 2. Aetiology of blindness

Meningitis	2
Usher's syndrome	2
Cataracts	2
Congenital	2
Still's disease	1
Behçet's disease	1
Retrolental fibroplasia	1
Tuberculosis	1
Cerebellar astrocytoma	1
Idiopathic	1

Reasons for Nonimplantation

Two patients had aidable hearing and are at present undergoing hearing aid trials. One patient at present awaiting surgey was initially aidable when first seen 4 years ago but no longer derives benefit from her aids. Three patients were offered implantation but either refused outright or else exhibited a very negative attitude to surgery. Two of them are still under review.

Results

Three of the four Nucleus patients are regular users, with open set speech discrimination and can converse on the telephone with people whose voices they know. A fourth patient became a nonuser.

Case 1. This 57-year-old man (fig. 1) is as good as the best of the sighted patients in the Manchester series. He had been blind from birth. He had a progressive hearing loss and had been totally deaf for 3 years prior to implantation. He acquired good open set discrimination within a week of switch on, and has continued to improve since (30 mFU). He converses naturally in a favorable environment with almost no use of finger spelling. He listens to the radio daily.

Case 2. This man of 60 was deaf for 14 years from Behçet's syndrome and from a failed stapedectomy. He had been blind from Behçet's syndrome for 40 years. He acquired immediate open set discrimination at switch on and has continued to improve (36 mFU). His ability to perform on standard testing is markedly worse than his observed ability to converse with members of his own family all of whom have a very strong regional

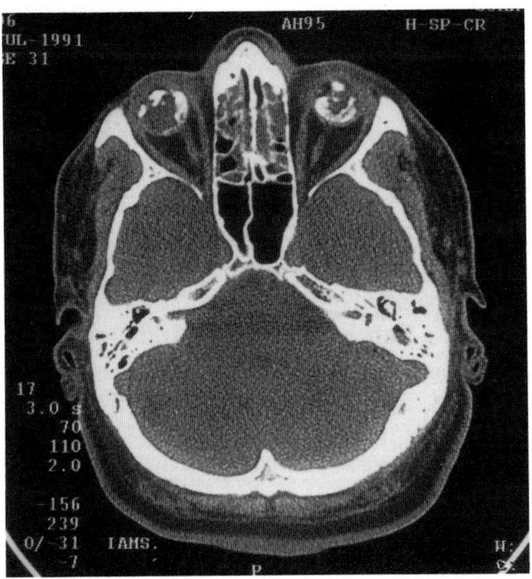

Fig. 1. CT scan showing typical ocular changes in retrolental fibroplasia.

accent. He was a jazz pianist prior to losing his hearing, and now derives some pleasure from playing the piano again.

Case 3. This 19-year-old girl lost both hearing and sight as a result of Still's disease: she has been totally deaf for 3 years and blind for 6 years. She was switched on recently (2 mFU) and is already beginning to converse on the telephone with her mother.

Case 4. This elderly lady of 81 used her device regularly for several months after switch on but had to abandon its use when, following an upper respiratory tract infection, she developed tinnitus in the implanted ear, which was exacerbated when the implant was switched on. She was the only nonuser in the whole Manchester series of 36 patients. She developed carcinoma of the oesophagus 18 months after implantation and has since died.

Case 5. This 63-year-old man lost his sight and vision at the age of 4 as a result of meningitis. It was felt that the most that a cochlear implant could offer would be some relief from auditory isolation, with little prospect of speech discrimination. For this reason and because there appeared to be some loss of cochlear patency on CT scanning, it was decided to refer him to Mr. J.G. Fraser at University College Hospital, London, where a single-channel extracochlear device was inserted. He is happy to have some perception of environmental sound but has no speech discrimination.

Discussion

The problems of rehabilitation of the deaf blind represent a unique challenge for the cochlear implant team. The disabilities that such dual sensory deprivations impose are impossible for the normally hearing and sighted community to comprehend. Although it is pointless to make comparisons between the handicaps, of the two, Helen Keller found deafness the greater affliction. She wrote:

'Deafness is a much worse misfortune. For it means the loss of the most vital stimulus – the sound of the voice that brings language, sets thoughts astir and keeps us in the intellectual company of man'.

The courage and cheerfulness with which the deaf blind face life is both humbling and moving. It is wrong to assume, however, that all deaf blind patients want to return to the world of sound and sight. The deaf blind culture has a strong identity which all do not necessarily want to leave. In this small series three potential implantees effectively refused the offer of an implant. One in particular holds a high position in the British deaf blind community. In addition, having carried out considerable research into cochlear implantation, he expressed a fear of a possible facial paralysis. It is important for the implant team to understand the role of the deaf blind culture in shaping decision making, and in this area the psychologist on the Manchester team has made a major contribution. It may be significant that in all 14 patients wishing to be assessed for implantation the duration of the deafness was considerably less than the blindness (mean of 14 years as compared with mean of 35 years). In other words these were all patients who had depended on hearing during years of blindness, and for whom loss of hearing was the final push into isolation. As yet there have been no patients referred who have lost vision after years of deafness.

Deaf blind people 'talk' to each other by means of finger spelling, they read one or more of the languages for the blind such as Braille or Moon, and they communicate at a distance using some form of electric transcription machine such as Hasicom. It is important that the team develop familiarity with these techniques and methods. The nurses who care for the patients during hospitalisation and the team who are involved with day-to-day rehabilitation develop these skills very rapidly. The national or local deaf blind associations will provide interpreters, but is important for the team to learn the skills for themselves. All test material has to be available in Braille or Moon and in this area too the blind and deaf blind organisations provide invaluable help. Rehabilitation and retuning sessions are naturally more time consuming than with sighted patients.

Three of the 4 patients who have received Nucleus 22-channel intracochlear devices have achieved good-to-excellent open set speech discrimination. One was obliged to stop using her device because of an increase in her tinnitus so her level of performance was impossible to assess. The decision to send the fifth patient for a single-channel device was based at least in part on the assumption that because of the perilingual onset of the deafness and its duration (59 years), he would be highly unlikely to achieve open set discrimination with a multichannel system, and the best he might expect would be a loss of auditory deprivation. The good quality of performance of the multichannel users leads one to speculate that the brain deprived of one sensory input (i.e. vision) can somehow use to better effect than others the relatively rudimentary auditory signals that it receives through the implant. This remains a matter of conjecture.

Conclusion

Multichannel cochlear implantation has a major part to play in the rehabilitation of certain deaf blind individuals, and these patients may be amongst the most worthwhile to consider for cochlear implantation. The implant team must acquire certain skills, and must not forget the strength of the cultural background from which these potential candidates come.

Acknowledgements

The authors are grateful to Mr. J.G. Fraser for allowing them to report on case 5.

This work is supported by two charities, HEAR, and Electronic Aids for the Blind. The authors gratefully acknowledge their invaluable assistance.

Richard T. Ramsden, FRCS,
Department of Otolaryngology and Centre for Audiology,
University of Manchester, Oxford Road, Manchester M13 9WL (UK)

Fraysse B, Deguine O (eds): Cochlear Implants: New Perspectives.
Adv Otorhinolaryngol. Basel, Karger, 1993, vol 48, pp 182–186

Ethical and Medicolegal Aspects of Multichannel Cochlear Implantation in Children

John J. Shea III, Elizabeth H. Domico

Shea Clinic, Memphis, Tenn., USA

Information about the Counseling Tool

Families begin and go through the process of obtaining a cochlear implant for their child with a set of expectations. If unrealistic or inappropriate, these expectations can negatively affect their perceptions of the child's progress following surgery and can cause the child to resent the implant if undue pressure is put upon him to succeed.

The pediatric cochlear implant team must take responsibility to ensure that families possess appropriate expectations. To that end, preoperative counseling plays a vital role in the selection process. Additionally, the continuation of counseling postoperatively is an important component of rehabilitation.

Various counseling tools, such as true-false tests, questionnaires, and attitude scales are available to aid the counseling process and have been used in our pediatric implant program. After hearing repeatedly issues of common concern to the families in our program, we began using a counseling aid which combines these issues with elements of existing tests.

Our test is administered after the parents have made an initial commitment to pursue implantation, and then again just prior to surgery. The test is presented as a series of statements which can be answered 'true', 'false', 'don't know', or 'not applicable'. Following completion of the test and regardless of the answer, we counsel about each statement to provide reinforcement or correction. The test form and the answer key plus all notations are filed in the patient's permanent medical record.

Specific areas are addressed by the test and are as follows.

Speech Perception

Families of postlinguistically deafened children may expect at least limited open-set recognition of connected speech material depending on duration of deafness prior to implantation, electrode insertion length, and other factors. Benefits to congenitally and perilinguistically deafened children may vary depending on age at implantation and other demographic factors, will develop slowly over time, and may not match those of postlinguistically deafened patients. The long-term development of benefits for these children remains to be discovered.

Use of Visual Cues

Lipreading skills may improve following implantation and training. If the child uses sign language as part of his communication mode, he may or may not reduce his reliance upon them. Parents whose children have developed language through total communication need to understand that signs are an integral part of the child's understanding of his world. To desire or expect cessation of signing after implantation is unfair and unrealistic and, furthermore, may cause the child to infer that something is wrong with him.

Environmental Sounds

The cochlear implant will allow the child detection of many environmental sounds. Training will be needed, however, before the child learns to recognize and associate meaning with these sounds. Many parents have stated that they will be happy even if the only benefit which the implant provides is the ability to hear a danger signal, such as a car horn. Families need to understand that to perceive a sound, recognize it, and respond to it appropriately comprise a complicated series of steps and may take some time for the child to develop.

Perception of Voices

The implanted child will be able to hear other people's voices as well as his own. Families need to be reminded that the ability to 'hear' a voice is not synonymous with 'understanding' what was said. Most families have been told from other sources that voices sound 'robotic' or like 'Donald

Duck'. Many fear that their child will sound like this when he talks following implantation. The dynamics of the vocal tract need to be discussed with the family to allay their apprehensions.

Speech Production

In our clinical experience, the main benefit parents hope the child will receive from implantation is the ability to develop speech. We have found that what parents mean by this is the ability to develop normal speech and language just like the hearing members of the family. Analysis of the speech samples of congenitally and perilinguistically deafened children to date suggests that while the underlying elements of speech become more understandable following implantation and training, the intelligibility of connected speech is slow to follow. For the postlinguistically deafened child, the cochlear implant will enable him to more easily monitor his speech and may retard and even reverse negative changes in speech production that occurred following the hearing loss.

Academics

Some families look to implantation as a guarantor of their child's success academically. If the child is in a hearing-impaired classroom, parents may expect that mainstreaming will suddenly be easy for the child. Counseling regarding the influence of a variety of factors besides hearing acuity on a child's educational advancement is necessary to address these perceptions. Certainly, the contribution of the implant team's deaf educator is of particular benefit here.

Special Services

Cochlear implantation does not automatically mean that services, such as interpreting, note-taking, resource room, speech therapy, and auditory training will be no longer be necessary. Indeed, the contribution of the latter two to the child's rehabilitation cannot be emphasized enough.

Postoperative Rehabilitation

Many parents view cochlear implantation as an end in and of itself, rather than a means to an end. Counseling regarding the necessity of training by a professional to help the child learn to make use of the new sounds auditorally and in speech is very important. In addition, the role of the parent in providing a home environment which fosters listening and speech development needs to be stressed. Finally parents need to understand their role in ensuring that the professionals working with the child at school and/or in private therapy are providing him with the training he needs. The cochlear implant team can make recommendations, but it is the parents' responsibility to make sure that adequate therapy is provided.

Interpersonal Relationships

Expectations about the impact of cochlear implantation upon a child's relationship with parents and others are often unrealistic. The teenage candidate may have concerns about 'fitting in' with his peers and fear that the implant will make him seem different. The desire to blend with a peer group is strong at this age and may be detrimental to rehabilitation with the device. The responses of the teenager to this part of the test must be carefully considered and given serious weight in the final decision to offer implantation.

Parents of congenitally and perilinguistically deafened children may expect that implantation will allow their child to function with ease in the hearing society and that deaf culture will no longer be of importance to the child. Parents of children with behavioral problems may believe that improved hearing will result in improved behavior without any other changes needed in the dynamic of the parent-child relationship. While the desire to make a child as 'normal' as possible is understandable, it is an inappropriate and unrealistic goal for cochlear implantation. It is in this area especially that we have found the services of our implant team psychologist to be invaluable.

Recreational Activities

Parents have expressed concern that cochlear implantation may curtail the kind and amount of recreational activities enjoyed by the child. The issue of head injury and the potential for harm to the internal portion of the receiver should be addressed.

Future Technology

Families should be counseled regarding the potential expense of future technology. Although efforts are made to upgrade software and external components of the implant system, thereby avoiding additional surgical procedures, these upgrades may not be provided free of charge.

Risks of Cochlear Implantation

Parents must be fully informed of the risks of the surgical procedure, the chance that the internal device may fail, and the possibility that the child may not successfully respond to electrical stimulation.

Parental Disappointment and Frustration

An important way to deal with and minimize unmet expectations is to adequately counsel the family preoperatively and continue this counseling aggressively following postoperative stimulation of the cochlear implant. The inclusion of the counseling tool in the patient's medical record is helpful since parents can be reminded of areas addressed preoperatively. In certain instances, the family may need to receive services from the team psychologist or a professional in their locality to deal with the changes that having an implanted child can bring to family relationships.

Another way to aid parents in adjusting to the realities of implantation is to put them in contact with other parents of implanted children. We insist upon this preoperatively and have found it to be helpful postoperatively as well.

John J. Shea III, MD, 6133 Poplar Pike, Memphis, TN 38119 (USA)

Fraysse B, Deguine O (eds): Cochlear Implants: New Perspectives.
Adv Otorhinolaryngol. Basel, Karger, 1993, vol 48, pp 187–190

Multichannel Cochlear Implantation in Prelingually and Postlingually Deaf Children

Alain S. Uziel[a], *Françoise Reuillard-Artières*[b], *Michel Mondain*[a], *Jean-Pierre Piron*[a], *Martine Sillon*[b], *Adrienne Vieu*[b]

[a] ENT Department, Hôpital Saint-Charles, Montpellier, France;
[b] Cochlear Implant Rehabilitation Center, Institut Saint-Pierre, Palavas-les-Flots, France

The management of children with cochlear implants represents a special challenge for the otologist. It is a complex area leading to many difficulties, requiring a wide variety of resources and expertise. One of the major requirements of a children's cochlear implant center is a multidisciplinary team [1–3]. Children referred to the Montpellier University Children's Cochlear Implant Center are seen by a team that includes two otologists, one audiologist, three speech pathologists, one educator of the hearing-impaired, one psychologist and hearing research scientists. The team takes in charge the candidate selection and preoperative assessment, the surgery, and the postoperative management including speech processor programming, training and evaluation. Our children cochlear implant center is located in a children's institute close to the Mediterranean seashore. The child and his mother come 3 days per month in the center for speech processor adjustment, training, and postoperative assessment of perceptual skills.

Patients and Methods

Between 1987 and 1992, Montpellier University Children Cochlear Implant Program has implanted 23 children: 13 under the age of 4 years, 6 from 6 to 10 years, and 4 from 10 to 13 years. Nine of them were congenitally deaf, 7 prelingually deaf, one was perilinguistic and six postlinguistic. A Nucleus 22-channel implant was used in 20 of the 23 children, and a 3M/House single-channel implant in 3 children. the etiology of deafness was: meningitis (6), viral infection (4), ototoxicity (1), hereditary (1), progressive hearing loss (1), Mondini malformation (1), and unknown/congenital (9). During the last 3 years, 48 children have been referred to the center for cochlear implantation. Twenty-three were selected for implantation. The selection criteria were the following: bilateral profound deafness, little benefit from a 6 month hearing aid trial, patent cochlea, auditory educational program, appropriate family motivations. Of the 16 congenitally and prelingually deafened children, 13 were implanted between 3 and 5 years of age, and 3 between 6 and 8 years. Of the 25 nonselected children, 11 had benefit from hearing aids, 9 were congenitally deaf children with more than 8 years' education with total communication, 4 had no family motivation, 1 had a Michel deformity.

The standard surgical procedure included an extended endaural incision, a simple mastoidectomy with facial recess approach. Partial ossification at the round window was found in 8 of 23 cases (34%). No total ossification was encountered in this series. A full insertion was completed in all the cases. All children were programmed with 20–22 electrodes, with a common ground electrode configuration. Electrically evoked stapedial reflex thresholds were determined peroperatively in order to predict the postoperative comfort levels.

An objective follow-up was done by recording every session with the speech pathologist on videotape. The assessment of speech perception skills was achieved using the tests selected by the European Children Implant Program: (1) phoneme detection (detection of presence or absence of sound); (2) perception of speech patterns (intensity and time speech cues); (3) closed-set word identification; (4) closed-set sentence identification; (5) open set speech recognition.

Results

Postlingually Deaf Children

Of the 6 postlingually deaf children, 4 had a short duration of deafness (<3 years). These children showed performance similar to those of adult implanted patients with open set word recognition at the 12-month follow-up. One of these children was previously implanted with a 3M/House single-channel implant, and was reimplanted 1 year later in the same ear with a Nucleus implant. This child showed remarkably rapid acquisition of auditory skills with a dramatic increase of open set word recognition from 0% using the 3M implant to 60 and 90% at the 1 and 9 months postoperative follow-up with the Nucleus implant. The two children with longer duration of deafness showed poorer results with open set word recognition not exceeding 20%.

Congenitally and Prelingually Deaf Children

A typical example of acquisition of perceptual skills in a congenitally and prelingually deaf child is given in figure 1. The congenitally deaf child could detect phonemes presented through the audition alone condition by

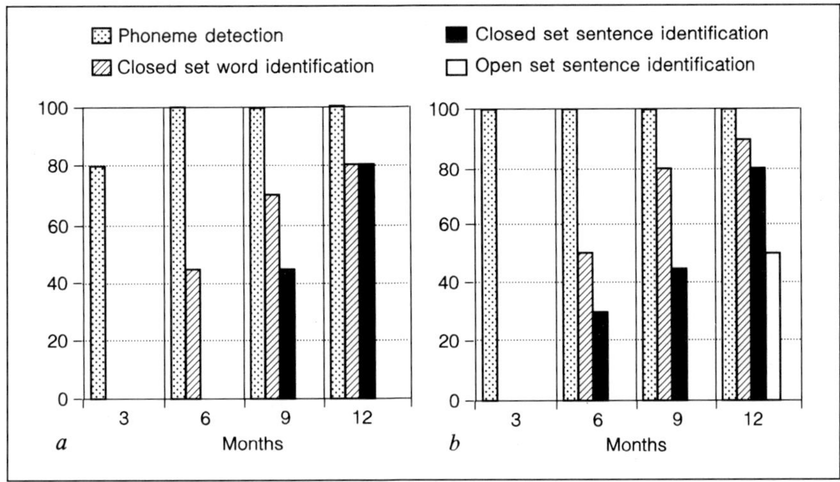

Fig. 1. Evolution of speech perception scores in a congenitally deaf child (*a:* duration of deafness = 2.9 years) and a prelingually deaf child (*b:* age at onset = 1.5 years; duration of deafness = 2.7 years).

the 3rd month of follow-up. By the 6th month, he could achieve spectral perception with word identification scores increasing from 40 to 80% at the 12th month of follow-up, and sentence identification scores increasing from 40% at the 9th month to 80% at the 12th month of follow-up. The acquisition of auditory perceptual skills is similar in the prelingually deaf child, except that he could achieve some open set recognition at the 12th month of follow-up.

On the 16 congenitally and prelingually deaf children, 50% could achieve speech pattern perception after 6 months' experience, 100% after 9 months. After 12 months' experience, 90% demonstrated closed set word and sentence identification, only 20% demonstrated open set speech recognition.

Conclusions

This study shows that prelingually and congenitally deaf children demonstrate clinically significant benefit across a broad spectrum of abilities after 12 months of follow-up with the Nucleus implant. However, training over a longer period of time is necessary to present the long-term results of Nucleus multichannel implants in children [4, 5], and to check for a difference between congenitally and prelingually deaf children. Our data suggest that early implantation is advisable in congenitally and prelingually deaf children since there may be a critical period [6] after which only minimal benefit is expected from cochlear implantation.

References

1 Clark GM, Blamey PJ, Busby BA, et al: A multiple-electrode intracochlear implant for children. Arch Otolaryngol Head Neck Surg 1987;113:825–828.

2 Hellman SA, Chute PM, Kretschmer RE, Nevins ME, Parisier SC, Thutston LC: The development of children's implant profile. ADD/Ref 1991;136:77–81.

3 Lehnhardt E: Experience with the Nucleus multichannel cochlear implant. Rev Laryngol 1991;112:343–346.

4 Staller SJ, Beiter AL, Brimacombe JA, Mecklenburg DJ, Arndt P: Pediatric performance with the Nucleus 22-channel cochlear implant system. Am J Otol 1991;12 (suppl):126–136.

5 Dowell RC, Dawson PW, Dettman SJ, et al: Multichannel cochlear implantation in children: A summary of current work at the University of Melbourne. Am J Otol 1991;12 (suppl):137–143.

6 Pujol R, Rebillard G: Experimental study of sound deprivation. Int Symp Cochlear Implants: New Perspectives, Toulouse, 1992, abstr 1, p 2.

Prof. Alain S. Uziel, MD, ENT Department, Hôpital Saint-Charles,
F–34059 Montpellier Cedex (France)

Fraysse B, Deguine O (eds): Cochlear Implants: New Perspectives.
Adv Otorhinolaryngol. Basel, Karger, 1993, vol 48, pp 191–198

Interactive Software for Setting Cochlear Implants in Children

D.J. Allum[a], *A. Mortlock*[b]

[a]Cavale International, Basel, Switzerland; [b]Cochlear Pty Ltd, Sydney, Australia

In response to the needs of clinicians, a software package has been specifically designed to aid fitting the Nucleus speech processor for children [1]. Programs have been created to test auditory perceptual skills [2] such as thresholds, balancing for either loudness or pitch, same-different tasks and loud-soft discrimination. The prototype programs are graphics-based, interactive and emphasize simple animations. They reward attention to auditory input whereas most other available software packages focus on stimulating speech output [3] or language development [4].

The aims of the routines are to increase the child's independent, active participation in the programming process and to reduce testing factors such as time needed to obtain behavioral responses, the number of professionals involved and the general expenses associated with fitting a cochlear implant. Also they should reduce the need for 'adult explanations' of a task.

Further, clinicians are often faced with parents who interrupt the testing sessions or give too many clues about what they think their child should, or should not, be hearing. Clinicians may have difficulty interpreting a child's actions. Inexperienced clinicians may fail to change activities frequently or provide rapid reinforcement so that a child's interest is not maintained.

Frequent task change is especially important for children who do not understand how and why they should respond. The tasks should provide the clinician with the information needed to program the speech processor. For example, there are children who provide *no* behavioral responses, who lose interest rapidly, who become distracted or give inappropriate responses, or who are simply too compliant to provide a reliable indication of what is being heard. Problems with unreliable responses lead to incorrect hearing levels, either too high or in a range which is so soft that there is no loudness growth (a so-called long T-tail). There is thus a need to find reliable methods for eliciting clearer responses from children.

Although T-levels are relatively easy to measure, clinicians often spend too much effort attempting to obtain precise values. The process of obtaining them can be quite time consuming for the clinician and boring for both children and adults. T-levels are not the most critical for fitting the speech processor. Perhaps clinicians spend unproductive time on this task because of its importance in basic audiology and for hearing aid fitting. The interactive pediatric software is equipped with a wide variety of routines for obtaining T-levels and aims to reduce the time taken for this task.

For fitting the speech processor, obtaining C-levels is a far more critical task. It is difficult to obtain C-levels from young children, as well as from long-term and congenitally deafened subjects. The major problem is that the concept of 'maximum comfortable level' (C-level) is difficult to describe. Loudness growth to electrical stimulation does not increase linearly, at higher levels the growth is much more rapid. Children may find a signal which suddenly becomes too loud both surprising and unpleasant. To the inexperienced listener, who does not have a clear frame of reference for loud and soft, loudness is suddenly 'too much'. On the other hand, some children are not distressed by loud sounds because their lack of knowledge of what is 'too loud' simply makes it impossible to report the phenomenon. Thus, in some cases, very loud signals may be required in order to ensure that the signal is, in fact, too loud.

Such challenges led to the development and initial evaluation of some very basic graphics programs, resulting in some important findings. The screens needed to be simple, with no distracting background images and limited use of color. The first impulse was to make very interesting images, but the images became more exciting than the listening tasks. The variety of the pictures was more important than the complexity. It was also found that a minimum interval between the child's response time and the reward was necessary. Long animated sequences that do not require interaction from the child were less useful. Instructions needed to be simple and, if possible, self-explanatory. Probably the most significant lesson was that activities should not be so interesting that children become completely absorbed in the task and oblivious to the auditory stimulation delivered

Table 1. Psychophysical tasks

Skill		Task		Programming element
Detection	⟶	presence-absence	⟶	T-level
Identify maximum comfortable loudness	⟶	too much or comfortable	⟶	C-level
Balance for loudness	⟶	same/different soft-loud	⟶	equalize dynamic ranges
Place-pitch identification	⟶	same/different low-high	⟶	place-pitch order

The skill describes what is required of a child to indicate the perception of an auditory signal. The task describes what the child is taught to indicate. The programming elements relate specifically to features of the MAP which are applied through the speech processor to transmit auditory signals to the implant.

through the implant. The problem of creating graphics which are more absorbing than actually required is not new. In 1983, Harvey Long at IBM remarked on the 'graphics madness' used in some teaching software. He called this 'The Law of Diminishing Astonishment', i.e. people grow to dislike that which they enjoy at the beginning of a program, especially if the program is time-consuming and repetitious.

Four main questions should be answered when programming the speech processor: (1) At what value is a 100% response level obtained? (2) When does the child experience a sensation which is too loud or too much? (3) Are adjacent electrodes similar or equal in loudness? (4) Is there an identifiable difference between place-pitch electrodes?

Table 1 illustrates how simple tasks can answer complex questions. A complete MAP (mathematical look-up table used to convert acoustic signals into perceptual units) can be achieved using the information derived from answering the first two questions. Balancing adjacent electrodes is an advanced task, but very useful because it helps to describe loudness growth and, ultimately, relates to the relative amplitudes of various frequencies making up speech patterns. When electrodes are not balanced, speech sounds rough or unnatural. Finally, the ability to distinguish whether an electrode differs in pitch from another electrode is useful, although not essential, in predicting whether patients are obtaining discrete frequency information.

A series of mouse-operated responses were used in the development of routines appropriate to the four questions above. Although it was uncertain whether very young children would be able to use a mouse, it soon became clear that they were much more dexterous than most of the clinicians. They also learned the concepts very rapidly.

The simplest operation was to press just one button. The child hears a signal (threshold), presses the button and something happens on the screen. Many different images can appear in unpredictable positions on the screen. In a testing situation, this variety kept the child's attention for more than 40 presentations – which equates to a lot of blocks dropping in a bucket. Another example of using a single button press is for the child to fill a screen with images. In this case, children became determined to fill the screen completely. It was useful to have the screen scroll down so that the child could continue to make new rows. A further example is where the child presses the mouse button with each perceived sound so that a picture behind a curtain is gradually revealed. The picture can be changed so that it is not predictable. There are many similar tasks for T-level measurement which are simple and easy to perform for children as young as 3 years old.

Another use of the mouse is simply to hold down one button for as long as a signal is heard. In this case, there may be a clear *off* response rather than an *on* response. An example is where a curtain moves upward as long as the child holds the button. When the signal stops, the child stops pressing the button and the screen stops. Children did not continue holding the button down when there was no signal and learnt this use of the mouse very quickly (fig. 1).

Another mouse operation is pressing either the right or left button. The youngest children were able to perform this task when the buttons corresponded to the right and left halves of the screen. Same/different tasks, which can be used for loudness balancing or pitch testing, are most easily assessed using this operation. The side of the screen which is selected will flash as long as a button is depressed. Originally, the screen was split in half horizontally, but the children could not easily relate the horizontal halves to the mouse buttons. Pressing the right or left button to indicate up and down, rather than to choose a screen side is a possible way to test C-levels. The concept of higher meaning louder, however, was not easily understood by the youngest children. C-level responses require much

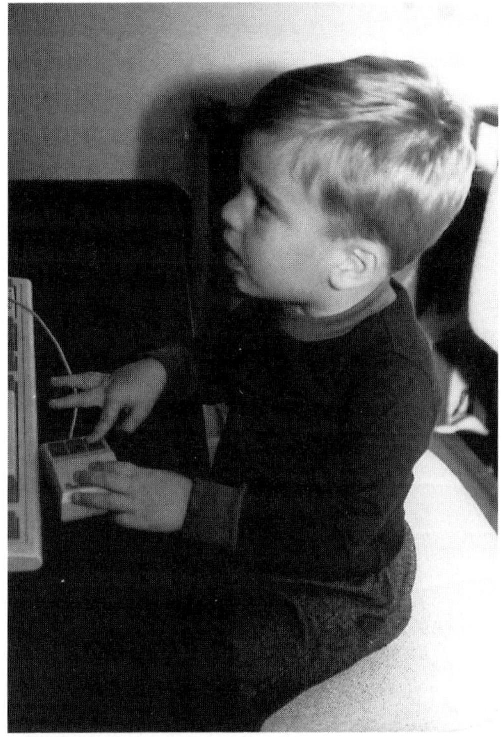

Fig. 1. This 2 years and 3 months old child is involved in one of the routines using right-left mouse buttons. He is choosing either right screen or left screen for a same-different task.

more training than T-level responses. An useful feature of the software is that it can aid in teaching the concept required to gain a response. With C-level testing, it was also found that the image used to reward a *too loud* response should not be so interesting that children go to that position simply to gain the reward.

A final operation is moving the mouse and selecting an image with a button push or moving the mouse while holding a button. Although these operations seem complex, 3-year-old children could do them. One particular task involved driving and parking a little car inside either a small or large garage by holding down a button and moving the mouse. The garages symbolised soft and loud. Here, a continuous signal which slowly increased

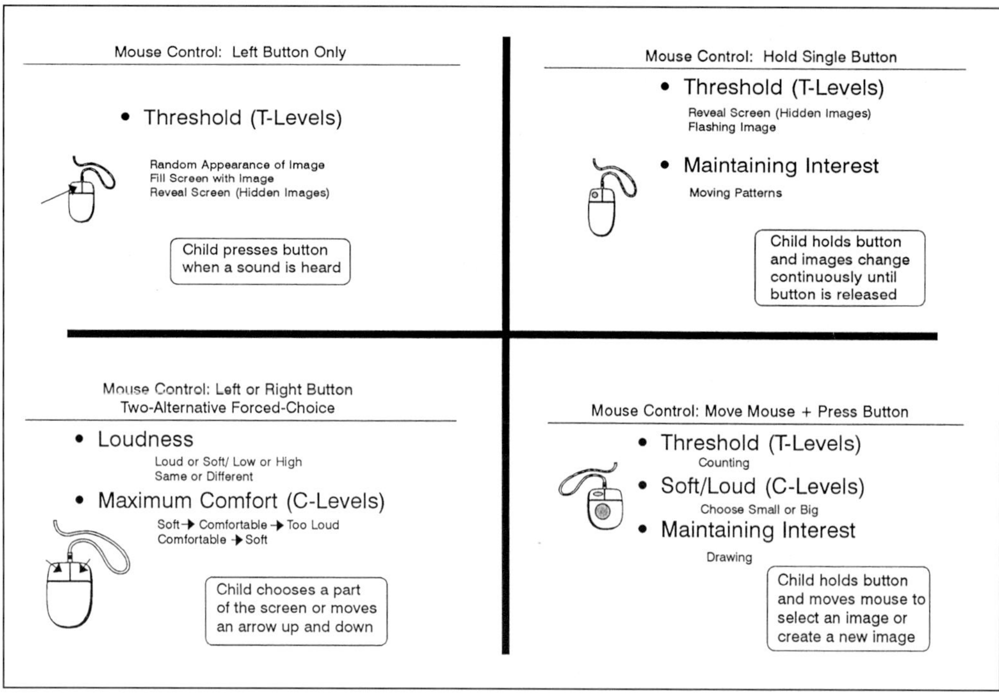

Fig. 2. Examples of the subroutines utilised in the trials. Different psychophysical tasks can be applied to the different mouse operations.

or decreased in loudness was used. It was possible to observe how the child perceived changing loudness as the car was moved from one position to the other. For a summary, see figure 2.

These and other programs were tested in a clinical trial conducted in four centers located in Australia, Germany, and Switzerland. Two separate computers with no physical connection were used where the stimulation from the standard Diagnostic and Programming System (DPS) software was not electrically synchronised with the screen actions. Audio output signalled the stimulation so clinicians could judge the accuracy of the children's responses. Thus, one computer was used with the normal DPS setup [1] and another computer was dedicated to the animated software (fig. 3).

The children tested were aged 3–8 years and randomly selected from those who were at a clinic during the trials. The experience of the clinicians

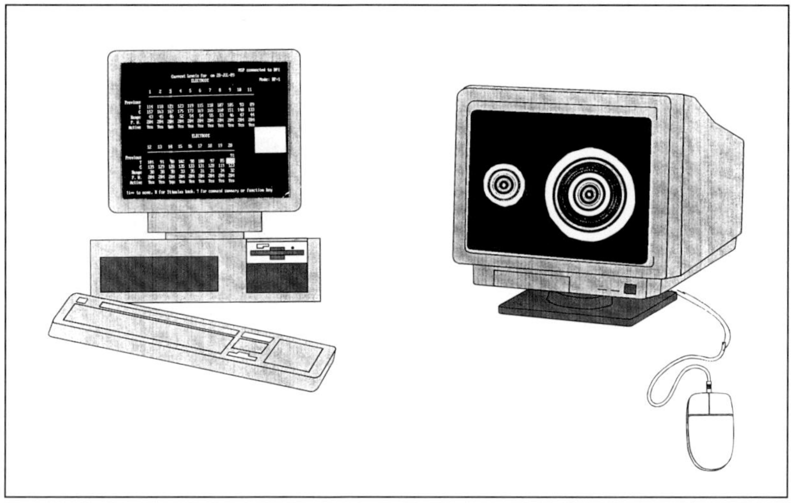

Fig. 3. Physical set-up of the hardware. Two separate computers were used. The computer supplied with the pediatric software was connected only to the mouse. The child did not have access to the keyboard. The DPS was used in its standard configuration.

ranged from average experience (2 or more children) to very experienced (10 or more children). The results revealed that all children learned to operate the mouse; attention span increased for all children, and with increased attention span, the number of electrodes that could be tested in one session increased; more reliable (repeatable) responses were obtained; clinicians spent less time changing games and maintaining the child's attention; and once the child learned the task, only one clinician was needed during the testing.

Children with an average attention span of 3–5 min were willing to sit in front of the monitor and cooperate with the testing for as long as 20–25 min. They waited patiently for routines to be changed and at the very least attempted the new tasks. As a button push or mouse movement resulted in some visual reward, the children did not become frustrated when they could not do the task perfectly and the clinician could quickly change to another routine.

These initial findings are very encouraging. The next phase is to develop more C-level tests. The trials have shown that it is best to avoid discrete steps for this task. Children tend to consider the task finished when all the steps on the screen have been accomplished, even if the C-level has not yet been measured. Finally, further work is being done to improve the graphics, increase the image options, and interface the software package with the already existing programming software available through Cochlear. The development of functional, effective software is a long process. It involves a number of interactions before it can be released for public use. It is hoped that this pediatric software will be available in the future to clinicians worldwide who work with children and the Nucleus device.

Acknowledgments

We would like to thank the Cochlear Implant Center (Hannover); Audiology Department, Kantonsspital (Basel); the Paediatric Cochlear Implant Programme (Nottingham); the Cochlear Implant Centre (Melbourne), and the Children's Cochlear Implant Centre (Sydney) for their comments and advice.

References

1 Beiter AL, Staller SJ, Dowel RC: Evaluation and device programming in children. Ear Hear 1991;12:25–33.
2 Osberger MJ: Auditory skill development in children with cochlear implants. Semin Hear 1986;7:423–432.
3 IBM: SpeechViewer. California, Peal Software, 1992.
4 Meyers L: Unique contributions of microcomputers to language intervention with handicapped children; in Meyers L (ed): Augmenting Language Skills with Microcomputers. Semin Speech Lang 1984;5.

Dr. D.J. Allum, Cavale International, Hebelstrasse 109,
CH–4056 Basel (Switzerland)

Fraysse B, Deguine O (eds): Cochlear Implants: New Perspectives.
Adv Otorhinolaryngol. Basel, Karger, 1993, vol 48, pp 199–202

Audiovisual Test Programs in Native Languages

Test Material in Norwegian on a Video Disc Controlled by Laser Bar Code

Erik Teig, Henrik H. Lindeman, Ole Tvete, Solveig Hanche-Olsen, Kjell Rasmussen

Department of Otolaryngology, Rikshospitalet, University of Oslo, Norway

Routine use of cochlear implantation in the treatment of profoundly or totally deaf patients has produced a need for standardized tests to evaluate the communicative skills before and after the operation with subsequent training. Based upon previous experience with tests using live voice with a known speaker, it was decided to adapt the contents of the Iowa video disc [1] to Norwegian and to extend the test material which could then be fitted in on the two sides of a standard video disc. The Iowa sentences are derived from the English BKB sentences [2]. The purpose of the present article is to give information on our test material for future reference and for audiological groups who might want to produce similar test material in other languages.

Production of Test Material

Ten medical students or young doctors, 5 females and 5 males, read all the test material which was recorded on a U-matic video tape. The TV screen showed the whole head and the open collar of the speaker. The regular sound was recorded on one track while a six-speaker babble was recorded on the other track. After reviewing the tape it was decided to use only 2 female and 2 male speakers. These speakers had the most consistent performance, and they varied between themselves both in speaking rapidity and in facial expression. One speaker spoke relatively slowly and was easy to lipread, while another speaker spoke relatively fast and was more difficult to lipread. The 2 others had speaking qualities in between. It was thus hoped to get a test which would cover a wide range of patient performance.

The selected taped test material was transferred onto a video disc which consists of:

(a) The Norwegian equivalents of the Iowa sentences [1] extended from the original 100 sentences to 120 sentences presented twice, with 60 sentences by each speaker.

(b) Norwegian translations/transcriptions of the Danish HELEN test [3], which is a series of simple questions to be answered with one word only. The test consists of 8 lists of 25 sentences. Each speaker presents 50 sentences.

(c) The consonant test where all 14 consonants + kj, sj, ng are presented in an a-consonant-a and in an i-consonant-i frame. The consonant test is thus very similar to the Iowa consonant test, but stress was put on the first syllable to make it sound more natural to the Norwegian ear. Each speaker presents each combination twice.

(d) The vowel test where the 9 Norwegian vowels are presented in a b-vowel-b frame. This produces nonsense words such as bib, bab, beb, and thus differs from the English h-vowel-d constellation where all combinations produce meaningful words. Again, each constellation is presented twice by each speaker.

Arrangement of Test Material into Lists

The laser video disc has the great advantage that the quality is constant and that any part of the disc can be accessed within a few seconds by the proper commands. This can be achieved by attaching the video disc player which must have a RS-232 interface to a laser bar code reader. Each test sentence or test utterance is identified on the disc by a laser bar time code, as shown in figure 1. By running the laser pen over the code, the corresponding sentence or utterance is presented on the screen. The laser bar codes have been made with the Mac WIT Bar program on a Macintosh PC.

IOWA-setninger, Liste 1
Resultat:
1
22140 - 22260
Vi har mye snø om vinteren.
2
38053 - 38176
Planten står i vinduet.
3
366 - 497
I hagen vokser det blomster.
4
12937 - 13075
Om høsten faller bladene av trærne.
5
24006 - 24160
Moren hørte at barnet skrek.

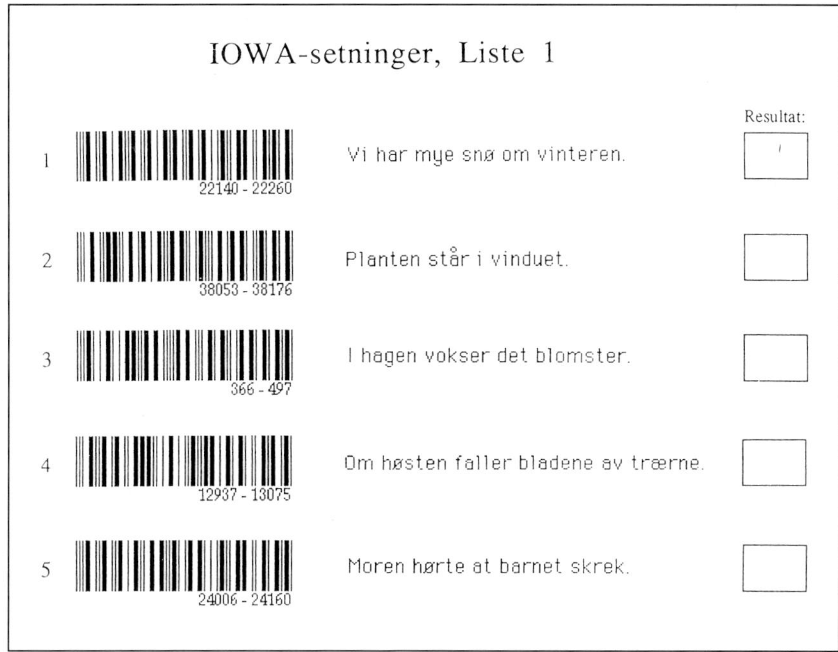

Fig. 1. Example of barcoding of test sentences as they appear on the test sheets.

We have chosen to arrange the Iowa sentences into lists of 20 sentences (= approximately 100 words), where each speaker presents 5 sentences. We wanted to use our tests in three situations, testing lipreading skills only (LO), hearing only (HO) and lipreading and hearing combined (LH) [4]. We also wanted to test each patient (1) before implantation; (2) after implantation and initial training; (3) at follow-up 3–12 months after implantation, and (4) 2–3 years after implantation. This requires 4 tests of 3 lists which equals 240 sentences. Since we only had 120 different sentences, we made 12 lists of 20 sentences where two sentences on each list were repeated on another list by another speaker of the opposite sex. This should make the training effect minimal.

The HELEN test lists with 25 questions composed in a special way related to colour, weekday, month, opposite of etc. was divided among the speakers in 6+6+6+7 sentences. Since a full test (LO, HO, LH) requires 75 questions, repetition over time must be accepted.

Presentation of Tests

We use a 20″ TV with two hifi speakers in a soundproof room. The test person is placed at a distance of 2 m from the TV screen, and the sound level at the site is approximately 65 dB SPL. So far, our system appears to be a convenient and useful tool for evaluating both potential cochlear implant candidates and implanted patients.

References

1 Tyler RS, Preece JP, Tye Murray N: Iowa Audiovisual Speech Perception Laser Videodisc. Iowa City, University of Iowa, 1987.
2 Bench J, Kowal A, Bamford JM: The BKB (Bamford-Kowal-Bench) sentence lists for partially hearing children. Br J Audiol 1979;13:108–112.
3 Ludvigsen C: Construction and evaluation of an audiovisual test (the Helen test). Scand Audiol 1974;(suppl 4):67–75.
4 Plant G, Macrae J: Testing visual and auditory visual speech perception; in Martin M (ed): Speech Audiometry. London, Taylor & Francis, 1987, pp 179–206.

Erik Teig, MD, PhD, Department of Otolaryngology, Rikshospitalet,
N–0027 Oslo (Norway)

Fraysse B, Deguine O (eds): Cochlear Implants: New Perspectives.
Adv Otorhinolaryngol. Basel, Karger, 1993, vol 48, pp 203–206

An Audiovisual Feature Test for Young Deaf Children in English, French, Spanish and German

Richard S. Tyler[a], *Gertrud Champe*[b]

[a]Departments of Otolaryngology – Head and Neck Surgery and Speech Pathology and Audiology, and [b]Department of Continuing Education: Translation Laboratory, University of Iowa, Iowa City, Iowa, USA

We have recently developed an audiovisual feature test in English for young deaf children [1]. This test has several attractive features and can easily be adapted for use in other languages. The purpose of this report is to describe the test and some of its advantages, and to make some preliminary suggestions about the use of similar test items that could be used in other languages.

The response form for this test is shown in figure 1. It is primarily based on the letters of the alphabet, which are often learned early in life by most children. Ross and Randolph [2] previously developed a speech perception test based on the entire alphabet. We selected only alphabet letters that could be presented in a consonant /i/ format, and included some additional words in the same format that would be familiar to a young deaf child and could be easily pictured.

Before the test begins, it is necessary to ensure that the children have the test items in their vocabulary, and associate the correct label to each of the test items. This is often accomplished by having a child label each of the test items, or having them point to the items in response to sign or a lipreading-only presentation. If a child does not know the items then the child cannot take the test at that time. Parents or teachers can be asked to practice the child on those items, and the child could then return at a later date.

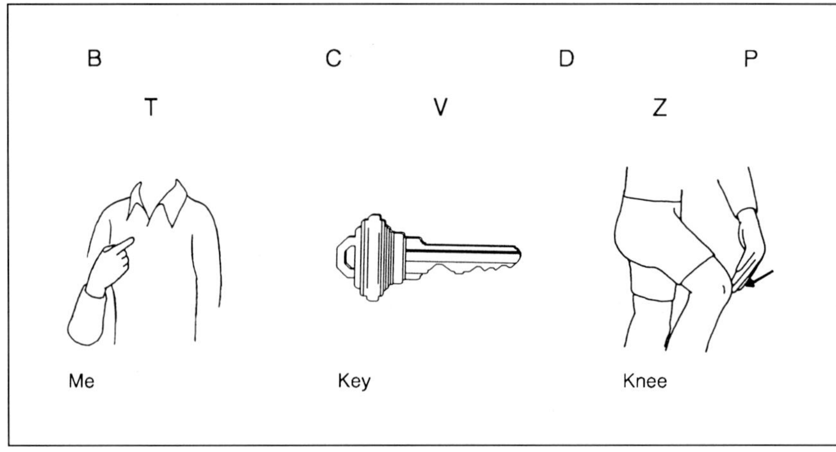

Fig. 1. Response form from the Audiovisual Feature Test in English. From Tyler et al. [1].

In the test, the child hears a single stimulus, for example /si/ and then points to the correct symbol 'C'. In our current application of the test, we present each item 6 times in random order, for a total of 60 stimuli per test. Additional stimuli could be presented to increase the test's reliability. If the child's limited attention does not permit the administration of all 60 stimuli, then a subset could be presented and combined with the results from another subset administered during another session.

This test has several advantages shared by other closed-set nonsense syllable tests, including the ability to: (1) evaluate the phonetic feature error patterns [3, 4]; (2) provide multiple presentations of the test without concern that becoming familiar with the test items will influence the results; (3) administer multiple lists that are equally difficult – this is particularly important in comparing performance across children or across audiovisual conditions.

In addition, this particular test is useful because it can be administered to many deaf children who are 5–6 years of age and older, something not possible with most nonsense syllable tests.

Preliminary results with this test are reported by Tyler [5] and Tyler et al. [6]. They reported that the phonetic errors committed by congenitally deafened children with cochlear implants were generally consistent with those committed by adult cochlear implant users. For example, the place of

Table 1. Preliminary recommendations for test stimuli to be used in different languages

Test phoneme	English	French	German	Spanish
/b/	b	b	b	b
/d/	d	d	d	d
/g/			g	
/p/	p	p	p	p
/t/	t	t	t	t
/k/	key	quai (warf)		¿que (what)
/f/		fée (fairy)	Fee (fairy)	
/v/	v	v	w	
/s/	c	c		
/z/	z		See (lake)	
/m/	me			
/n/	knee	nez (nose)	ne (no)	
/ts/			c	
/ð/ (voiced th)				c
/tʃ/ (ch)				ch
/ʒ/ ('zh') as in measure)		g		

In English, the stimuli are the test phoneme coupled with the vowel /i/. In the other languages, the stimuli are the test phoneme coupled with the vowel /e/. The English translation is shown when words are used in other languages.

articulation feature was poorly transmitted by the implant but was received well when lipread.

Table 1 presents some preliminary suggestions for the application of this test to other languages. Although the test will not be directly comparable across languages, it will allow speech features to be tested in young deaf children in these languages. As with the English-language version, letters or pictures that are not known by the child can be trained by the teacher or parent so that the child could be tested at a later date.

Conclusions

We have developed a speech feature test for young deaf children that has some important advantages for the appraisal of device efficacy and the planning and evaluation of rehabilitation. We are preparing additional versions of this test for use in other languages.

Acknowledgements

This work was supported in part by National Institute of Health Program Project Grants NS20466 and DC00242 and by grant RR59 from the General Clinical Research Centers Program, Division of Research Resources, NIH, and a grant from Lions Clubs of Iowa.

References

1 Tyler RS, Fryauf-Bertschy H, Kelsay D: Audiovisual Feature Test for Young Children. Iowa City, University of Iowa, 1989.

2 Ross M, Randolph K: A test of the auditory perception of alphabet letters for hearing-impaired children: The APAL Test. Volta Rev 1990;92:237–244.

3 Miller GA, Nicely PE: An analysis of perceptual confusions among some English consonants. J Acoust Soc Am 1955;27:338–352.

4 Wang MD, Bilger RC: Consonant confusions in noise: A study of perceptual features. J Acoust Soc Am 1973;54:1248–1266.

5 Tyler RS: What can we learn about hearing aids from cochlear implants. Ear Hear 1991;12(suppl 6):177S–186S.

6 Tyler RS, Opie J, Fryauf-Bertschy H, Gantz BJ: Future directions for cochlear implants. J Speech Lang Pathol Audiol 1992;16(2):151–164.

Richard S. Tyler, PhD, Department of Otolaryngology, University of Iowa,
200 Hawkins Drive E230 GH, Iowa City, IA 52242-1078 (USA)

Educational Setting for Children

Fraysse B, Deguine O (eds): Cochlear Implants: New Perspectives.
Adv Otorhinolaryngol. Basel, Karger, 1993, vol 48, pp 207–209

Long-Term Follow-Up of Nucleus Cochlear Implant Patients

C.-E. Rochette, J. Verville, L. Fortier

Département de Langues et Linguistique, Université Laval, Québec, Canada

Our specific objective is a tentative inside view of the linguistic and phonetic changes of a group of patients during a 24-month period after rehabilitation. We are interested in measuring the efficiency of oral communication due to cochlear implant. Evaluation is based on a phonetic and linguistic point of view.

Thirteen adult patients had regular hearing and listening training with the help of a Nucleus cochlear implant (65 intensive periods of 2 h based on an analytical to global approach learning program). From the results obtained during the 4 months' readaptation, 9 of these 13 patients were considered to make a homogeneous group.

We kept in contact with them during 2 years, by making them do evaluation tests at the 3rd, 6th, 12th, 18th and 24th months after rehabilitation. Our main questions: Do these patients improve or get worse during the 2 years of normal activities, following the end of their readaptation? What phonetic and linguistic elements are affected?

The tests applied were elaborated and validated beforehand with normal subjects as well as 7 deaf persons. Table 1 shows some goals of measurement in these tests as well as the number of phonetic and linguistic elements. A quick look will also let you see the evolution of results in percent for the whole group through the five sessions of evaluation.

To help you see the variations in relation with the nature of the linguistic test contents better, table 2 presents a global view of the evolution. It is detailed from the most important losses to the best effective improvements.

Table 1. Long-term follow-up results (%)

Linguistic elements	Number	Patients				
		1	2	3	4	5
Vowel discrimination	360	60.0	52.2	53.9	55.9	52.2
Consonant discrimination	252	90.5	85.7	83.3	86.5	88.5
Identification of monosyllables	180	33.9	23.9	28.9	30.6	29.4
Identification of dissyllables	220	27.3	25.0	31.7	35.6	22.2
Intonation	108	89.8	78.7	80.6	70.8	78.7
Localization of stress	135	91.9	94.8	97.0	91.7	96.3
Flow velocity	90	100.0	97.8	98.9	100.0	98.9
Rhythm (number of syllables)	220	91.4	86.4	75.0	74.5	71.8
Sentences – device	135	43.7	50.4	51.1	58.3	48.9
Sentences – lipreading	135	60.0	65.2	80.0	83.3	83.7
Sentences – device + lipreading	135	93.3	91.9	97.8	98.3	97.8
Differentiation of dissyllables	180	93.3	93.9	93.9	95.6	89.4
Timed reading	600	55.05	59.92	60.73	52.84	44.89
Identification of vowels	116	71.6	72.9	59.2	52.3	53.1
Identification of consonants	170	67.6	68.8	51.0	48.5	50.8

Table 2. Variations according to linguistic contents

Linguistic content	Gains and losses	Evaluation
Identification of vowels	–	. . . .
Rhythm (number of syllables)	–	. . . .
Identification of consonants	–	. . . . . .
Timed reading	–	. . . . . .
Intonation	–	. . . . .
Vowel discrimination	–	. . . . .
Identification of dissyllables	–	. . . .
Differentiation of dissyllables	–	. . . .
Identification of monosyllables	–	. .
Consonant discrimination	–	. .
Flow velocity	–	.
Accent	+	.
Sentences – device	+	. . .
Sentences – device + lipreading	+	. . . .
Sentences – lipreading	+	. . . . . .

What are the main observations?

(1) Note that 11 of the 15 analyzed linguistic elements show maximum to minimum regression (identification of vowels to rate of utterances) and these changes occur mainly during the last 6 months of the follow-up period.

(2) Only four linguistic aspects that we examined show an improvement in performance during the same last 6 months: identification of accent, understanding of sentences with the implant device only, sentences with the device and visual support (mainly lipreading) and sentence recognition with lipreading only.

(3) These specific improvements concern mainly the most common linguistic units in languages (sentences) to the detriment of detailed or isolated units (syllables, sounds and words, etc.).

(4) Sentences with lipreading are the element that improved most.

What do we learn from these results?

The hearing training program insisted mainly on the fundamental units like phonemes (consonants and vowels), syllables and isolated words to help patients stabilize the phonological system based on new signals. The sentences through conversation or different real experiences, that make the natural set of communication, were not neglected. Everyone knows that sentences play a major role in communication. Here they improved, obviously because of the daily usage of the cochlear implant, without the necessity of hearing all the minute phonetic units that set up sentences.

Our common language use is similar to that of the implanted patients: we decode messages by first recognizing all that is mostly significant, usually group of words; and then, if necessary, we will listen to details (syllabification in oral language and spelling in written language) from time to time. We can even go further in guessing the missing details without processing to precise phonetic analysis of an oral message.

These results stress that the biggest change occurred in lipreading sentence improvement! We would have thought that improvement in hearing would have made the implanted patients take less and less advantages of the visual support, which means in their case, lipreading. In fact, in spite of the benefits of 2 years' use of the cochlear implant, they did not fully change their listening and hearing habits or, at least, they went back to their previous attitude easily. This seems to be confirmed by a detailed analysis of the results in relation with the duration of deafness: the longer the deafness, the fastest they go back to lipreading.

Dr. C.-E. Rochette, Département de Langues et Linguistique, Université Laval, Québec G1K 7P4 (Canada)

Fraysse B, Deguine O (eds): Cochlear Implants: New Perspectives.
Adv Otorhinolaryngol. Basel, Karger, 1993, vol 48, pp 210–215

Cochlear Implants in Adolescents[1]

Patricia M. Chute

Cochlear Implant Center, Manhattan Eye, Ear and Throat Hospital,
New York, N.Y., USA

Cochlear implants is the state of the art in the treatment of children with profound deafness who do not respond with conventional amplification. In the nationwide study of 142 children, Staller et al. [1] reported that all children implanted showed significant improvements in the detection and discrimination of sound. Approximately half of these children obtained some open set speech recognition. Children who are post-linguistically deafened tended to be better performers. However, Staller noted that 16.3% of the pre-linguistically deafened children also achieved in a similar fashion. These children tended to be implanted at very early ages thereby sustaining shorter durations of deafness. However, the congenitally deafened adolescent implant user represents a competely different group of children since they have been deafened for more than 10–12 years. The limited benefits of auditory electrical stimulation on the speech perception abilities of these children should be viewed realistically in an effort to better counsel and select the appropriate adolescent for a cochlear implant.

The present study is a result of retrospective review of teenage implant patients followed by the Manhatten Eye, Ear & Throat Hospital Cochlear Implant Center. The subjects consisted of 10 teenagers who had 11 surgeries. Six children were implanted with the 3M/House device and 5 with the Nucleus 22 channel. One of the teenagers suffered a 3M/House internal receiver failure after 2 years and subsequently had a second surgery to insert a Nucleus device.

[1] Funded by the Children's Hearing Institute.

Table 1. Demographics

Age at implant	$\overline{X}$ = 14.9 years (range 13–19)
Duration of deafness	$\overline{X}$ = 13.8 years (range 10–16)
Mode of communication	7 TC 3 oral
Educational setting	6 mainstreamed 2 self-contained 2 school for deaf

Table 1 displays the demographic information for these children.

All the children except one Nucleus and one 3M/House were congenitally or pre/perilinguistically deafened. Test results at the pre-implant stage were compared with 1-year and 2-year postimplant use. Several of the children had data for longer periods, i.e. up to 5 years but interestingly enough there was very little difference in the results after the 2-year point. The data of 1 teenager, a Nucleus user, who had used the device for only 6 months has been included in the review.

In an effort to assess benefits obtained from both 3M/House and Nucleus 22 devices, the pre/post data were examined by selecting those tests that were common to both implant protocols, i.e. the Discrimination After Training Test (DAT) [2] and the Test of Auditory Comprehension (TAC) [3]. Both of these tests consist of closed set responses. The results of these tests are shown in tables 2 and 3.

Using the DAT, preoperatively the majority of the subjects scored at level 2 while 4 of the subjects were at levels 5 and 9, respectively. These 4 subjects (those scoring at levels 5 and 9 on the DAT) were implanted with the Nucleus 22 channel device. Postoperatively, the teenagers implanted with the Nucleus device performed at levels 11 and 12 while the remainder tended to perform at levels 7–9.

Results of the Test of Auditory Comprehension are reflected in table 3. Preoperatively 8 of the subjects were unable to pass level 1 of the TAC.

Postoperatively 3 subjects were still unable to pass level 1 at the 1- and 2-year intervals. The teenager that made the most gains was the postlinguistically deafened teen with the Nucleus device.

Table 2. Discrimination after training (DAT); n = 10

Preoperation	1 year after	2 years after
$\overline{X} = 4.4$	$\overline{X} = 8.2$	$\overline{X} = 9.6$
(2–9)	(5–11)	(7–12)

Table 3. Test of auditory comprehension (TAC); n = 10

Preoperation	1 year after	2 years after
X = 0.2	$\overline{X} = 1.2$	$\overline{X} = 1.5$
(0–2)	(0–3)	(0–5)[1]

[1] High score reflects the performance of post-linguistically deafened teen with Nucleus device.

Lipreading enhancement scores were difficult to pool since the test materials varied. The teenagers showed a relatively small degree of enhancement (<5%) with the exception of the postlinguistically deafened Nucleus user. This 1 subject displayed a consistent 10–12% enhancement across all testing intervals. Interestingly, however, in all cases where there was sufficient data it was found that as the lipreading plus audition scores increased, so did lipreading alone scores.

Although the Nucleus users received a wider variety of tests (these included portions of the Minimal Auditory Capabilities Test (MAC), Speech Patterns Contrast (SPAC), IOWA Battery and Three Interval Forced Choice Test (THRIFT)), assessment of benefit using these results was difficult since multiple revisions of the protocol during the early stages of clinical trials truncated some of the test procedures. On the average, however, there was a tendency for performance to improve slightly on the THRIFT in duration, vowel height and final consonant voicing. The performance on the remainder of the subtests was similar at the intervals measured.

In the light of these findings, it would appear that the majority of teenagers in this study gained minimally from the use of their implants as measured on this specific battery of tests. Some of these results become more understandable when the hours of implant use is investigated. Of the 10 teenagers, 4 are nonusers, 5 are full-time users and 1 is a limited user (2–4 h per day). The 4 nonusers were implanted with the single-channel device and were some of our earliest implant patients. The 1 limited user was the single-channel device failure who freely chose to opt for the second surgery to receive a multichannel device. The remaining 5 included one 3M/House and 4 Nucleus users. These teens wear their devices for 12–15 h daily and feel they are unable to function as well when they are without it.

Since the magnitude of benefit adolescents obtain with cochlear implants appears to be small based on current quantitative methods and instruments of assessment, it is important to note that the more successful users report definite qualitative enhancement in their lives. These teenagers have consciously and enthusiastically chosen to have and wear an implant. This fact needs to be recognized and further investigated through other methods. These may include those ethnographic measures made via direct interview and participant observation as well as speechreading under more degraded conditions. Additionally, given these data and observation, it becomes crucial that this population be carefully selected.

In an attempt to develop a program for teenage selection and follow-up, the Cochlear Implant Center at Manhattan Eye, Ear and Throat Hospital established a five-stage program to assist teenagers and their parents in making a decision regarding cochlear implant surgery. This program was developed after studying the profiles of both the nonusers and the full-time users to determine what factors needed to be addressed at the preoperative stage. This program known simply as TEENS includes the following components: Training; Education; Expectations assessment; Networking; School support.

Initially, all teenagers considering a cochlear implant are placed in formal training situations. Oftentimes this is done with vibrotactile stimulation. This accomplishes two things. First, it helps the teenagers realize that they will once again be in speech and auditory therapy that will require a significant time commitment. This priority is dramatically emphasized in real terms once they are placed in the position of actually having to give up part of their free time to participate in this essential therapy. Second, by wearing a vibrotactile device the cosmetics of wearing a body pack can be explored as well as their performance with this type of sensory aid.

The second stage is an educational process for the adolescent concerning all aspects of cochlear implant performance and surgery. Issues involving the surgery (especially the amount of hair shaved, the size of the bandage, hairwashing postoperatively and length of stay in the hospital) are carefully reviewed. The responses of their peers (both deaf and hearing) are also explored.

Stage three involves the assessment of the teenagers and their parents' expectations. Written responses are elicited to allow the candidates an opportunity to clearly list what they believe the advantages and disadvantages to the surgery will be. Expectations regarding speech production changes are discussed in great detail since this is often a secondary goal that is not directly stated by the adolescent.

The fourth stage involves networking the teenagers with other teenagers who have already been implanted. This is done using the TDD, written correspondences and in the majority of cases in a face-to-face meeting. Initially, the teenagers are introduced with the parent and audiologist present and then later with only the audiologist and finally with the teenagers alone.

The fifth and final stage incorporates the school guidance counsellor or psychologist as a valued resource. At the onset of the program, the teenager is placed in counselling which continues until at least 6–9 weeks postimplant. In some cases, it may continue on an on-going basis depending on the adolescent's needs.

Only after completion of these stages is a final decision made regarding the individual teenager's candidacy for an implant. This process takes place over at least a 6-month period and is carefully outlined at the time of the initial visit. Needless to say, teenagers who are not motivated or who are unrealistic rarely complete the program. For those that continue, the educational consultant and the audiologist monitor the process.

The overall results of cochlear implants in the teenage population appear to be similar to the pre-perilinguistically deafened adult [4]. For both groups the implant users progress from category I (using Moog and Geers classification) of no pattern perception to Category II – pattern perception [5]. The test scores for this group are at best disappointing. However, it is apparent that the present evaluation methods fall short in assessing the true benefits obtained from the device. Regardless, however, it behooves all teams implanting children to assess teenage candidates in a much more intensive manner in order to ensure the proper selection of the appropriate candidate.

References

1 Staller SJ, Dowell RC, Beiter AL, Brimacombe JA: Perceptual abilities of children with the Nucleus 22-channel cochlear implant. Ear Hear 1991;12(4 suppl):34S–47S.
2 Thielemeir MA: The Discrimination After Training Test. Los Angeles, House Ear Institute, 1984.
3 Office of Los Angeles County Superintendent of Schools. Test of Auditory Comprehension. North Hollywood, Foreworks, 1980.
4 Parisier SC, Chute PM: Cochlear implants: Indications and technology. Med Clin North Am 1991;75:1267–1276.
5 Geers AE, Moog JS: Predicting Spoken Language Acquisition in Profoundly Deaf Children. J Speech Hear Disord 1987;30:1–11.

Patricia M. Chute, MA, Cochlear Implant Center, Manhattan Eye, Ear and Throat Hospital, 210 East 64th Street, New York, NY 10021 (USA)

Fraysse B, Deguine O (eds): Cochlear Implants: New Perspectives.
Adv Otorhinolaryngol. Basel, Karger, 1993, vol 48, pp 216–221

Curricula Objectives for Educators of Children with Cochlear Implants

Kathleen C. Vergara, D.K. Oller, Rebecca Eilers, Thomas Balkany

University of Miami, School of Medicine, Mailman Center for Child Development, Department of Pediatrics, Miami, Fla., USA

The University of Miami in cooperation with Dade County Public Schools has developed a model program for investigating the use of sensory aids (hearing aids, tactile aids, and more recently cochlear implants) with hearing-impaired children. The program provides a comprehensive educational and therapeutic curriculum from the initial stages of diagnosis through the middle school level.

The program is located at the University of Miami Mailman Center for Child Development and at several Dade County Public Schools. The University-based program includes parent-infant, toddler, preschool, kindergarten and primary classrooms. The transition to the public schools is made when the students are prepared to enter elementary school mainstream programs in selected subjects. There, educators of the hearing impaired coordinate individualized educational programs that emphasize placing each student in the mainstream. Curriculum has been developed to incorporate auditory and speech training into the classroom while implementing conventional academic curricula.

When the United States Food and Drug Administration approved the use of cochlear implants in children with profound hearing impairments in June of 1990, the University of Miami initiated a cochlear implant program. Educators, audiologists and speech pathologists from the model program became members of the University of Miami's cochlear implant team establishing a strong link between the implant candidate's educational and medical centers. The cooperation of the members of this interdisciplinary team has provided optimal conditions for implant success with children from the model program.

Several other established pediatric cochlear implant teams use educational consultants whose responsibility is to be an advocate for the implant candidate and establish mutual rapport between members of the implant team, the family and educational professionals [1, 2]. The teachers and speech pathologists of the University of Miami model program assume this responsibility. They contribute valuable information about the implant candidate's educational progress and auditory awareness in the classroom, in therapy and at home during the selection, programming and rehabilitation process.

Evaluation Procedures

Each child enrolled in the program is given speech perception and production evaluations at 6-month intervals allowing progress to be monitored. These evaluations provide the implant team with data for determining implant candidacy and post-implant follow-up. The evaluation battery consists of tests using closed-set and open-set formats designed to assess auditory detection, discrimination, recognition and comprehension skills. The closed-set tests that are part of the battery are the Ling Five Sound Test [3], the Early Speech Perception Test [4], the Screening Inventory of Perception Skills [5], the Change/No Change Test [6], the Northwestern University Children's Perception of Speech Test [7], the Pediatric Speech Intelligibility Test [8], the Monosyllable-Trochee-Spondee Test [9], the Minimal Pairs Test [10], and the Common Phrases Test [5]. Other tests include the PBK-50 word lists [11], an open-set test, which is administered if the child is able to participate in this level of testing; Connected Discourse Tracking [12] which evaluates a child's ability to perceive conversational speech; the CID Phonetic Inventory [13]; and the Speech Pattern Contrast Test [14]. Speech production is evaluated by collecting audiotaped samples of the child's vocalizations.

The information provided by the test battery enables teachers to plan educational programs that will meet academic expectations as well as incorporate cochlear implant training and speech stimulation activities.

The philosophy of the model program is that auditory and speech skill development are essential ingredients of a hearing-impaired child's educational environment.

Cochlear Implant Goals and Objectives

Existing auditory training programs may be described [15] as analytic, with extensive training in the discrimination of syllables and contrastive auditory patterns, or synthetic, with concentration on training with phrases and sentences, and are appropriate for use with cochlear implant recipients. The Auditory Skills Curriculum [16], the Developmental Approach to Successful Listening [17], and Auditory Training [18] are examples of widely accepted curricula for auditory training.

Teachers and clinicians at the University of Miami Model Program have developed a hierachy of cochlear implant goals and objectives to integrate rehabilitation into the educational setting. The hierachy of goals is (1) *awareness of implant stimulation* with objectives that progress from device acceptance to detection; (2) *identification of auditory patterns* with objectives that progress from detection to recognition of auditory patterns in closed-set format; (3) *identification of suprasegmental patterns* with objectives that progress from awareness to recognition of duration, rate, intensity, pitch, stress and syllables in a closed-set format; (4) *identification of segmental auditory patterns* with objectives that progress from recognition of maximally contrastive phonemes and words to recognition of minimally contrastive phonemes and words in a closed-set format; (5) *identification of words and phrases* with objectives that progress from recognition of words to recognition of phrases in closed sets; (6) *tracking connected discourse* with objectives that progress from tracking preschool level stories to tracking advanced level stories; and (7) *generalization* with objectives that expand auditory recognition skills into familiar and unfamiliar settings.

The presentation of activities is related to the order of goals and objectives. Traditional auditory training programs require the accomplishment of a predetermined criterion before the child can move to the next objective. The design of this cochlear implant training program provides professionals with the freedom to establish their own criterion levels and to target various goals and objectives that match the child's abilities and interests. For word discrimination, a 12-month post-implant preschooler may need a criterion level of 25% accuracy while a 30-month post-implant preschooler may need a criterion level of 60% accuracy. When a specific criterion has been mastered, a higher criterion is established for the objective, but a child may progress to higher level objectives without total mastery of lower level criteria. Our clinical observations combined with results collected from the test battery given at six-month intervals suggest that a child's perception and production skills gradually improve over time in each goal category. Other recent research studies of children using cochlear implants also indicate improvement over time [5, 19, 20]. Consistent training in all goal categories is important to maximize the auditory potential of children using cochlear implants which will, in turn, enhance implant users' self-esteem [21].

Total Communication and Cochlear Implant Training

If children who use cochlear implants are to be successful, their teachers need to incorporate auditory training into the curriculum. This will encourage the use of audition to facilitate communication through speech. The University of Miami model program uses Non-simultaneous Total Communication [22] in which sign language functions as a bridge for the development of oral language skills with decreasing use of sign as the child's oral language skills become proficient. Academic training modules emphasizing oral communication are planned several times during each school day and are expanded as the child's skills improve. The success of this approach is based on the expectation that the child be an active oral participant.

Conclusion

Cochlear implants in children are raising concerns about the education of the hearing impaired. Auditory training once was considered to be an essential component of all educational programs, but with the introduction of total communication this philosphy changed. The advent of cochlear implants, tactile aids, and improved amplification has renewed interest in auditory training. As a result the development of listening skills is once again considered to be a fundamental ingredient in the education of hearing-impaired children.

References

1 Nevins ME, Kretschmer RE, Chute PM, Wellman SA, Darisier SC: The role of an educational consultant in a pediatric cochlear implant program. Volta Rev 1991;93: 197–204.

2 Kileny PR, Kemink JL, Zimmerman-Phillips S: Cochlear implants in children. Am J Otol 1991;12:144–146.

3 Ling D: Auditory coding and recording: An analysis of auditory training procedures for hearing impaired children; in Ross M, Giolas T (eds): Auditory Management of Hearing-Impaired Children. Baltimore, University Park Press, 1978, pp 181–218.

4 Moog JS, Geers AE: Early Speech Perception Test for Profoundly Hearing Impaired Children. St Louis, Central Institute for the Deaf, 1990.

5 Osberger MJ, Miyamoto RT, Zimmerman-Phillips S, Kemink J, Stroer B, Firszt J, Novak M: Independent evaluation of speech perception abilities of children with Nucleus 22 channel cochlear implant system. Ear Hear 1991;12(suppl):66S–80S.

6 Robbins AM, Osberger MJ, Miyamoto RT, Renshaw JJ, Carney AE: Longitudinal study of speech perception by children with cochlear implants and tactile aids: Progress report. J Acad Rehab Aud 1989;21:11–28.

7 Elliott LL, Katz DR: Northwestern University Children's Perception of Speech (NU-CHIPS). St Louis, Auditec, 1980.

8 Jerger S, Lewis S, Hawkins J, Jerger J: Pediatrics speech intelligibility test. I. Generation of test materials. Int J Ped Otorhinol 1980;2:217–230.

9 Erber NP, Alencewicz CM: Audiologic evaluation of deaf children. J Speech Hear Disord 1976;41:256–267.

10 Robbins AM, Renshaw JJ, Miyamoto RT, Osberger MJ, Pope ML: Minimal Pairs Test. Indianapolis, School of Medicine, 1988.

11 Haskins H: A phonetically balanced test of speech discrimination for children; unpublished master's thesis. Northwestern University, Evanston, 1949.

12 DeFilippo AL, Scott BL: A method for training and evaluating the reception of ongoing speech. J Acoust Soc Am 1978;63:1186–1192.

13 Moog JS: CID Phonetic Inventory. St Louis, Central Institute for the Deaf, 1988.

14 Boothroyd A: Evaluation of speech production of the hearing impaired: Some benefits of forced-choice testing. J Speech Hear Res 1985;28:185–196.

15 Osberger MJ: Audition. Volta Rev 1990;92:34–53.

16 Office of Los Angeles, California Superintendent of Schools, Auditory Skills Curriculum – Audiological Services – Southwest School for the Hearing Impaired. Foreworks, North Hollywood, 1980.

17 Stout GG, Windle J: Developmental Approach to Successful Listening (DASL). Houston, Houston School for Deaf Children, 1986.

18 Erber NP: Auditory Training. Washington, Alexander Graham Bell Association for the Deaf, 1982.

19 Dawson PW, Blamey PJ, Rowland LC, Dettman SJ, Clarke FM, Busby PA, Brown AM, Dowell RC, Rickards FW: Cochlear implants in children, adolescents, and pre-linguistically deafened adults: Speech perception. J Speech Hear Res 1992;35: 401–417.

20 Miyamoto RT, Osberger MJ, Robbins AJ, Renshaw J, Myres WA, Kessler K, Pope ML: Comparison of sensory aids in deaf children. Ann Otol Rhinol Laryngol 1989; 98:2–7.

21 Balkany TJ: An overview of the electronic cochlear prosthesis: Clinical and research considerations. Otolaryngol Clin North Am 1982;16:209–215.

22 Oller DK: A new age in education of deaf children: Methodological innovations and artificial hearing; in Wolraich M, Routh DK (eds): Advances in Developmental and Behavioral Pediatrics. London, Jessica Kingsley, 1990, vol 9, pp 161–180.

Kathleen C. Vergara, MA, University of Miami, School of Medicine,
Mailman Center for Child Development (D-820), Department of Pediatrics,
1601 N.W. 12th Avenue, Miami, FL 33101 (USA)

Results in Children

Fraysse B, Deguine O (eds): Cochlear Implants: New Perspectives.
Adv Otorhinolaryngol. Basel, Karger, 1993, vol 48, pp 222–230

Results in Patients with Congenital Profound Hearing Loss with Intracochlear Multichannel Implants

M.J. Manrique, A. Huarte, J.C. Amor, P. Baptista, R. Garcia-Tapia

Clinica Universitaria de Navarra, Departamento de Otorrinolaringología, Pamplona, España

In 1989 we began our cochlear implant program and to this moment we have performed 42 implants using the Mini Nucleus 22 channel cochlear implant.

Most of the patients, when we began, were postlinguistic, but in 1990 we started implanting 2 prelinguistic patients and during 1991 and 1992, 16 more.

Study of the Implant Population

In this work we studied a total of 15 patients with a congenital profound hearing loss, in which we consider 3 prelinguistic patients that lost their hearing in the first 6 months of life.

There were 4 males and 14 females, with a mean age of 16.55 years (SD 8.79); minimum and maximum of 6 and 38 years, respectively. We recognize the importance of performing the implant as early as possible, although it is difficult in our country. However, as we will see, although there are many late implants the results are satisfactory.

In table 1, we classify the patients by age groups and show aspects like etiology, use of hearing aids, sex, communication mode and length of insertion of the electrode array.

Table 1. Patient classification

	<15 years	>14 years	Total
Age, years	9.88	23.22	16.55
Sex			
Male	2	2	4 (22)
Female	7	7	14 (78)
Etiology			
Genetic	4 (44.4)	2 (22.2)	6 (33)
Prenatal infection	2 (22.2)	1 (11.1)	3 (17)
Ototoxicity	0	1 (11.1)	1 (7)
Postnatal infection	2 (22.2)	1 (11.1)	3 (17)
Unknown	1 (11.1)	4 (44.4)	5 (28)
Communication mode			
Oral	9 (100)	7 (77.8)	16 (89)
Total	0	2 (22.2)	2 (11)
Hearing aids	8 (88.9)	6 (66.7)	14 (78)
Length of insertion, mm	22.74	22.56	22.65
n	9	9	18

Percent values are shown in parentheses.

Table 2. Phonoaudiology study protocol

Audiologic explorations	Voice-language exploration
Pure tone audiometry	Voice study
Closed-set test	Fundamental frequency
Vowel recognition	Timbre
Consonant recognition	Phonatory rhythm
Series of words	Intonation
Sentences	Intensity
Open-set test	Language study
Bisyllabic test (Spondee recognition test)	Manchester scale
Monosyllabic test (PBK)	Gael-P test (children)
Sentences with clue	Spreen-Benton test (children)
Sentences without clue (CID sentences)	
Prosodic test (MACI)	
Lipreading test	

Method

One of our main objectives when we developed a cochlear implant program was the creation of a Phono-Audiological Protocol in Spanish.

We classified the audiological test into three groups: closed-set, open-set and prosodic. We have added to these tests pure tone audiometry in open field and lipreading. In table 2, we can appreciate the tests that form these groups. In parentheses, are those tests performed that are similar to the English-language test. It is obvious that we cannot speak of a total similarity, due to the differences between both languages.

In relation to the analysis of voice, at this moment we are performing more extensive studies. We will inform what has been observed with the fundamental frequency (Fo).

Results

Follow-up time ranged between zero and 2 years. Thirteen patients have worn their implants for more than 6 months, 5 patients for 1 year and 1 for 2 years. The results in these prelinguistic patients should be considered as preliminary due to the short follow-up period.

Pure Tone Audiometry

Auditory thresholds registered in frequencies that ranged between 500 and 4,000 Hz (fig. 1) did not vary significantly in the follow-ups performed during the first year, with mean values ranging between 53 and 55 dB HL. No differences were seen either between the two age groups of more than 14 years and less than 15 years.

Closed-Set

Considering the whole group of implanted patients, the results in vowel and sentences test show a statistically significant progression at 6 months and 1 year of evolution (table 3). The consonant recognition test was significant ($p < 0.01$) at 1 year of evolution. With this test a clear continuous progression was seen, especially when compared to results performed at 6 months.

As we analyze the results reached at 6 months, no significant differences between the two age groups were seen.

Open-Set

Global results (table 4) demonstrate the existence of a favorable progression for the monosyllable and sentence test with and without clues. The results were not statistically significant in any of the tests performed

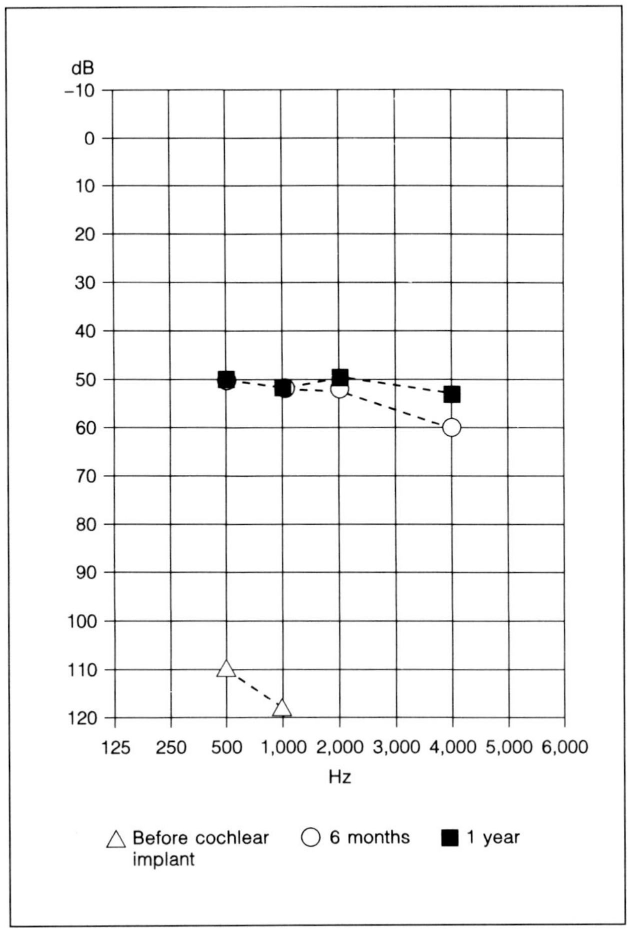

Fig. 1. Auditory thresholds in pure tone audiometry.

between either age groups. Patients of 15 years or younger had better results in the bisyllable and monosyllable tests and lower values in the sentences with and without clues tests.

Prosodic

Of the diverse prosodic aspects of the language, pronunciation was analyzed with this test.

Table 3. Closed-set

	Before cochlear implant			6 months after			1 year after		2 years after	
	<15 years	>14 years	total	<15 years	>14 years	total	<15 years	>14 years	<15 years	>14 years
Vowels	8.55	17.55	13.05	56.35	37.66	48*	–	52*	–	69
Consonants	3.44	0.44	1.94	9.2	7.33	8.18	–	15.2**	–	31
Sentences	16.66	28	21.62	72.85	81.6	76.5*	–	82.2*	–	75
n	9	9	18	7	6	13	0	5	0	1

* $p < 0.001$; ** $p < 0.01$.

Table 4. Open-set

	Before cochlear implant			6 months after			1 year after		2 years after	
	<15 years	>14 years	total	<15 years	>14 years	total	<15 years	>14 years	<15 years	>14 years
Bisyllabic	2	4.77	3.38	6.25	1.33	3.33	–	1.6	–	0
Monosyllabic	3.33	0	1.76	27.33	10.83	16.33*	–	19.6	–	0
Sentence with clue	2.77	2.85	2.81	3.33	13.33	8.33	–	20	–	25
Sentence without clue	0	0	0	0	4.5	2.25	–	3.4	–	0
n	9	9	18	7	6	13	0	5	0	1

* $p < 0.1$.

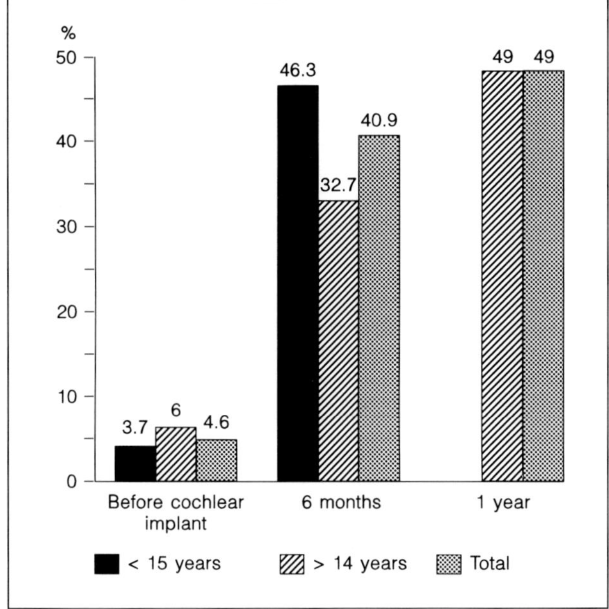

Fig. 2. Results of prosodic aspects of the language.

The results reached were very high (fig. 2) at 41 and 49% at 6 and 12 months, respectively ($p < 0.001$). These differences between 6 and 12 months were not significant, but a progression in time was seen. Better results were seen in the group of patients of less than 15 years, when these tests were performed at 6 months' follow-up.

Fundamental Frequency

An almost significant drop in the Fo ($p < 0.1$) was seen as it varied from 260 to 207.66 Hz at 1 year of evolution (fig. 3). This change was also evident in both age groups, with a tendency to a lower Fo.

Lipreading

Lipreading did not vary significantly during the first year of follow-up. Although the use of the cochlear implant provided better results, significant differences were not reached (fig. 4).

3
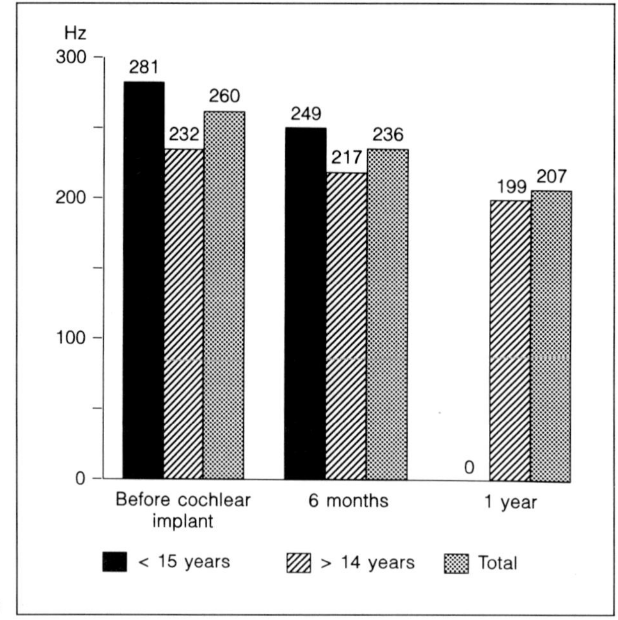

4
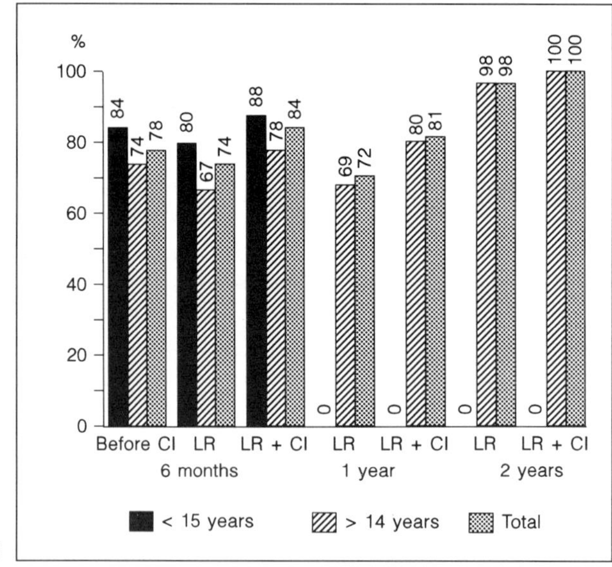

Fig. 3. Fundamental frequency.

Fig. 4. No significant differences during the first year of follow-up in lipreading (LR). CI = Cochlear implant.

Discussion

Unfortunately, the short period of follow-up of less than 1 year in our patients with congenital deafness can only provide provisional results. Time and the correct postimplant rehabilitation are important factors.

Nevertheless, the results obtained allow us to make various considerations. Attending to thresholds in the pure tone audiometry, no variations are seen in time. This may speak in favor of the absence of neuronal deterioration after 1 year of continuous stimulation with the cochlear implant. Other aspects that should be considered are the results obtained over the speech frequencies. This reflects the capacity of tonotopic stimulation that is provided by the implant.

In all closed-set tests a good outcome was seen, reaching very good results in the first 6 months in the vowel (48%) and sentence recognition (76.5%) tests. It was especially interesting to observe the increasing tendency towards improvement in the consonant recognition test; there was a regular and continuous rise during the first year.

The results in the open-set test did not rise above 20% in any case at the end of the first year. These results in absolute terms are poor, but we believe that they adjust to those of other authors [1–4]. The evolution referred in these patients by authors allow us to think of better results with time. As a fact, an evident progression during the first year is observed in the monosyllable and sentence test with clues. We believe that prudence should be kept in mind when offering expectations related to the acquisition of understanding the spoken word. Lipreading is fundamental to reach an adequate level of communication.

No differences were seen between both age groups at 6 months post-implantation. The scarce amount of patients at the 1-year follow-up in the group aged less than 15 years prevented us from analyzing if this will continue with time. Therefore, we will have to wait and see in the future how these results compare with those of other authors [5], in which there were more younger patients.

Special attention should be paid to the good results registered in the prosodic test in which favorable progress could be seen with time. We believe that this prosodic information provides an important contribution to voice and language.

The restoration of auditory-linguistic feedback through the cochlear implant is most responsible for the notorious change seen during the first year in the voice and to a lesser degree in language. We believe that one of the major benefits that the cochlear implant provides in congenital prelinguistic deaf patients is a better oral expression of language.

References

1 Staller SJ, Dowel RC, Beiter AL, Brimacombe JA: Perceptual abilities of children with the Nucleus 22-channel cochlear implant. Ear Hear 1991;12:34–47.

2 Tyler RS: Speech perception with the Nucleus cochlear implant in children trained with the auditory/verbal approach. Ann J Otol 1990;11:99–117.

3 Gantz BJ, Tyler RS, Knudson JF, Woodworth G, Abbas P, McCabe BF, Hinrichs J, Tye-Murray N, Lansing C, Kuk F, Brown C: Evaluation of five different cochlear implant designs: Audiologic assessment and predictors of performance. Laryngoscope 1988;98:1100–1106.

4 Isberger MJ, Robbins AM, Miyamoto RT, Berry JW, Myres WA, Kessler KK, Pope ML: Speech perception abilities of children with cochlear implants, tactile aids on hearing aids. Ann J Otol 1991;12(suppl):105–116.

5 Staller SJ, Beiter AL, Brimacombe JA, Mecklenburg DJ, Arndt P: Pediatric performance with the Nucleus 22 channel cochlear implant system. Am J Otol 1991; 12(suppl):126–136.

Dr. Manuel J. Manrique, Clinica Universitaria de Navarra, Departamento de Otorrinolaringología, Apartado 192, E–31080 Pamplona (Spain)

Fraysse B, Deguine O (eds): Cochlear Implants: New Perspectives.
Adv Otorhinolaryngol. Basel, Karger, 1993, vol 48, pp 231–235

Preliminary Speech Perception Results for Children with the 22-Electrode Melbourne/Cochlear Hearing Prosthesis

R.S.C. Cowan, R.C. Dowell, B.C. Pyman, S.J. Dettman, P.W. Dawson, G. Rance, E.J. Barker, J.Z. Sarant, G.M. Clark

Human Communication Research Centre, University of Melbourne;
The Australian Bionic Ear and Hearing Research Institute, and The Cochlear Implant Clinic, Royal Victorian Eye and Ear Hospital, Melbourne, Australia

The 22-electrode cochlear prosthesis developed by the University of Melbourne and Cochlear Pty Ltd. has been shown to provide significant speech perception benefits to profoundly deafened adults [1]. More recently, use of an improved Multipeak encoding strategy has significantly improved speech perception performance both in quiet and in noise [2, 3]. Benefits to speech perception in children have not as yet been fully documented, in part due to the shorter history of implant use in children and the smaller overall number of children implanted as compared with adults.

The first implantation of the 22-electrode cochlear prosthesis in a child was carried out in Melbourne in January of 1985. In Melbourne, a 5-year-old child was operated on in April 1986, and a first congenitally deaf child in April 1987. The age of implantation has been progressively reduced, with the first 2-year-old child implanted in Melbourne in 1990. As at January 1992, approximately 1,200 children (under 18 years of age inclusive) have been implanted worldwide with the 22-electrode cochlear prosthesis. Of this number, approximately 50% are under the age of 6 years.

The age of the child, aetiology of the hearing loss, age at onset and duration of the hearing loss, education program attended both prior to and subsequent to implantation, and parental motivation to assist in habilitation are all factors which may affect an individual child's development and progress with the device. Evaluation of performance in children is complicated by a number of issues, including the effects of delayed speech and language development, and the ability of individual children to perform auditory tests. The measure of performance chosen for any evaluation will also reflect the interests of the particular clinician, for example, effects of device use on speech production may be of interest to the speech therapist, whereas educational progress will be of primary importance to the teacher of an implanted child. However, in choosing an appropriate evaluation test to measure progress with the cochlear prosthesis, it is vital to realize that all measures such as effects of device use on speech production, educational progress, development of language, and effects on social and communication skills depend on the child being able to accurately perceive speech information through her/his device.

Method

Speech perception test results are collected preoperatively and postoperatively in the Melbourne programme. These results serve a number of purposes, including: (1) establishing that the speech processor is functioning properly and is properly mapped; (2) establishing speech perception, speech production and language goals for use in the habilitation programme; (3) establishing postoperative versus preoperative benefits for the child; (4) monitoring continuing improvements in performance over time.

While results of individual tests may be useful for any of these purposes, they are not as appropriate for evaluation of overall performance in groups of children, since the effects of factors such as age, and level of linguistic development cannot be readily controlled. In addition, the importance of patient factors such as duration of profound deafness, experience with the device, or educational placement cannot readily be assessed from individual test results.

In order to address the issue of differing linguistic development and age of children in the programme, a series of six stages or categories of speech perception were established. The individual categories are hierarchically arranged from 1 to 6, and include performance at the levels described as follows: (1) detection of speech sounds including high frequency consonants; (2) discrimination of suprasegmental features of speech, plus 1; (3) discrimination and recognition of vowel sounds, plus 1 and 2; (4) discrimination and recognition of consonant sounds, plus 1, 2, and 3; (5) open-set speech recognition with scores less than 20% for unfamiliar material, plus 1, 2, 3 and 4; (6) open-set speech recognition with scores greater than 20% for unfamiliar material, plus 1, 2, 3, 4 and 5.

These categories were used to analyze speech perception results for 40 children and adolescents implanted with the 22-electrode cochlear prosthesis.

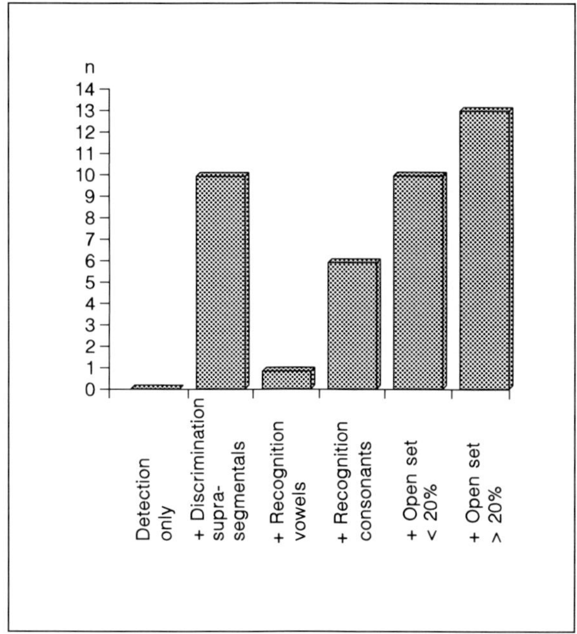

Fig. 1. Speech perception category achieved by implanted children (n = 40).

Results

Aetiology of hearing impairment varied across the 40 children and adolescents. A breakdown of hearing loss for the children showed that 24 of the children had congenital hearing losses (resulting from a number of specific aetiologies including: Usher's syndrome – 3, rubella – 2, CMV – 1, idiopathic – 8) versus 16 of the children with an acquired hearing loss (including meningitis – 11, progressive – 3, idiopathic – 2).

In all but 3 cases, the children were using 15 or more electrodes from the array in their programmed map. Of the 3 cases with less than 15 electrodes, 2 had an aetiology of meningitis and one had a congenital.

Figure 1 shows the number of children achieving speech perception results in each of the six speech perception categories. As shown, all children achieve a minimum of category 2 (discrimination of suprasegmentals). In total, 23 of the children, or 58% are in categories 5 and 6, indicating some open-set speech perception benefits. A total of 13 children, or 33% are in category 6, indicating open-set implant-alone speech perception scores of greater than 20% on unfamiliar material.

Discussion

While this is preliminary data only, a number of interesting findings are evident. First, the majority of children in the programme have a hearing loss due to congenital aetiologies rather than to acquired. This may reflect the epidemiological patterns in Australia and/or the patient selection strategies employed. However, the result differs from the previously held view that the majority of children in cochlear implant programs would have hearing loss due to meningitis.

Previous results with adults [4] have established that the number of electrodes used was a significant factor in predicting scores on sentence perception tests. Analysis of the patient details for the children shows that 37 of the 40 children are using 15 or more electrodes. Although adult data can only be applied cautiously to children, the results suggest that the majority of the children would have enough electrodes for adequate speech perception.

The division of the 40 children into the six speech perception categories showed a number of points. First, no child is achieving only at the level of category 1 (detection of speech sounds). As shown, 58% of the children are achieving some open-set speech perception, placing them in categories 5 and 6. Analysis of contributing factors showed that the majority of children achieving categories 5 and 6 have used the cochlear prosthesis for periods longer than 1 year, and had periods of profound deafness less than seven years prior to implantation. At present, the majority of children in category 2 are those children who have used the device for less than one year. This is encouraging, since it suggests that many of the children currently achieving at the level of category 2 may also reach the open-set levels of category 5 and 6 with additional experience with the device.

More detailed statistical analysis of the results will examine the interaction of speech perception category with a number of factor including duration of profound deafness prior to implantation, number of years of experience with the device, educational placement of the child, age at implant, and residual hearing levels prior to implantation. This analysis will identify factors important in predicting potential benefits from the device for individual children, and will assist in preoperative counselling and recommendations to parents.

References

1 Dowell RC, Mecklenburg DJ, Clark GM: Speech recognition results for 40 multichannel cochlear implant patients in the USA and Australia. Arch Otolaryngol 1986; 112:1054–1059.

2 Dowell RC, Whitford LA, Seligman PM, Franz BH-K, Clark GM: Preliminary results with a miniature speech processor for the 22-electrode Melbourne/Cochlear hearing prosthesis. Proc XIV World Congr Otorhinolaryngology, Head and Neck Surgery, Madrid, September 1989. Amsterdam, Kugler & Ghedini, 1990, pp 1167–1173.

3 Skinner MW, Holden LK, Holden TA, Dowell RC, Seligman PM, Brimacombe JA, Beiter AL: Performance of postlinguistically deaf adults with the wearable speech processor (WSP III) and mini speech processor (MSP) of the Nucleus multi-electrode cochlear implant. Ear Hear 1991;12:3–22.

4 Blamey PJ, Pyman BC, Gordon M, Clark GM, Brown AM, Dowell RC, Hollow RD: Factors predicting postoperative sentence scores in postlinguistically deaf adult cochlear implant patients. Ann Otol Rhinol Laryngol 1992;101:342–348.

Dr. R.S.C. Cowan, Australian Bionic Ear and Hearing Research Institute,
384 Albert Street, East Melbourne, Vic. 3002 (Australia)

Fraysse B, Deguine O (eds): Cochlear Implants: New Perspectives.
Adv Otorhinolaryngol. Basel, Karger, 1993, vol 48, pp 236–240

Total Obstructed Cochlea and Cochlear Implant

C.H. Chouard, B. Meyer, N. Garabedian, K. Dupuch, C. Fugain, L. Monneron

ENT Department, Hôpital St-Antoine, Paris, France

In the case of total obstructed cochlea (total ossification or osteofibrous total obstruction) the electrodes array of the multichannel device Minisystem-22 from Cochlear must be placed in a large (0.7 mm) and deep well dug in the cochlea. This partial placement is always responsible for either total failure or at least severe dysfunction of the implant. On the contrary, the easy introduction of the electrode of the single-channel Monosonic from MXM in a small (0.125 mm) cochlear well supplies the patient with a constant and non-negligible speech understanding, which is directly due to its recent [1] sound-processing improvement. The multichannel failure is due to the too small number of functional electrodes. In order to know if it is reasonable to try and place this electrode array, we studied the minimal length of this array to be introduced, i.e. the minimal number of functional electrodes which are necessary to obtain a speech intelligibility superior to those provided by the MXM single-channel device.

Material and Methods

Intelligibility Performances Assessment

This comparative study has been based on the intelligibility without lipreading of 4 parameters: (1) vowel and consonant discrimination obtained by 118 pair presentations (in these tests, the random response is 50%); (2) closed lists of 10 homosyllabic sentences, and (3) half-open lists sentences.

Patients

We studied the results of 7 patients suffering from acquired deafness implanted with the Nucleus device, successively lighting off the 19 first electrodes, then the 17 first electrodes, and then the 15 first electrodes having, respectively, only 3, then 5, then 7 functional electrodes. We compared these successive performances with the obtained results on 8 patients suffering from acquired or congenital deafness, implanted with a Monosonic (table 1) using their implant daily for at least 3 weeks. On the Cochlear device array the mean length of an electrode and its silastic ring is about 0.75 mm around the tip of the array. For each patient and each possibility, we selected the best strategy, which happened in all cases to be common ground and multipeak.

Results

The results are described in figure 1. We may observe that with 7 functional electrodes, the efficacy of the multichannel system is superior to that of the monochannel system. The corresponding length of the electrode array is around 5.4 mm.

Discussion

These experiments were elicited on the one hand by the double failures which we encountered trying to implant a multiple electrode array in 2 cases of total ossified cochlea, and, on the other hand, the clinical results we obtained in 11 patients (7 young children and 4 adults) presenting with total obstructed cochlea owing to the single-channel system from MXM and its new digital speech signal processing.

Comparison of the patients' performances must be discussed first. On the one hand, one may observe that the multichannel group had been placed in an acute situation, without any apprenticeship, whereas the single-channel group performances were assessed after at least 3 weeks of daily use. But on the other hand, one may underline that among the 8 single-channel patients 2 presented with totally ossified cochlea and 4 were prelingually deaf adults or teenagers, who generally achieve poor clinical results; on the contrary, the multichannel group was represented by adults suffering from recently acquired deafness. And precisely, the least satisfactory results are generally obtained when the etiology of deafness is congenital or prelingual.

The superiority of the Cochlear device on the MXM device appears if all the 7 last electrodes of its array are functional. That is probably due to the fact that the Nucleus speech-coding strategy is used almost normally in these cases. On the contrary, if there are only 5 functional electrodes – that is the best possibility in our experience if this device is used in the case of

Table 1. Clinical status of the patients studied

Monosonic								
Patient/sex	Mor/F	Bal/M	Cha/F	Gri/F	Thu/F	Dut/M	Hou/M	Dai/M
Date of birth	7/10/27	28/5/43	26/9/41	15/8/34	19/5/81	27/3/74	21/11/70	25/12/73
Age when deaf	22	42	47	47	3	3	2	0
Etiology	mumps	skull fracture	meningitis	chronic otitis	meningitis	meningitis	strepto-mycin	maternal rubella
Date implanted	16/12/87	26/5/88	11/10/89	24/1/90	21/7/89	9/8/89	14/6/90	13/11/90
Age implanted	60	45	48	54	8	15	19	16
Duration of deafness	38	3	1	7	5	12	17	16
Remark			ossified cochlea		ossified cochlea			
Functional electrodes	1	1	1	1	1	1	1	1
Minisystem-22								
Patient/sex	Tos/M	Sul/F	Bal/M	Bal/M	Leo/M	Chas/F	Dec/M	
Date of birth	31/4/64	13/2/39	28/5/43	13/4/55	20/11/28	26/9/41	26/11/58	
Age when deaf	26	32	45	35	20	47	33	
Etiology	Kogan	progressive deafness	skull fracture	otosclerosis	tuberc. meningitis	meningitis	vascular	
Date implanted	5/12/91	15/5/91	25/9/90	8/1/92	11/4/91	5/12/91	9/1/92	
Age implanted	27	42	47	37	62	50	34	
Duration of deafness	1	10	2	2	42	3	1	
Remark						partially obstructed cochlea		
Functional electrodes	19	16	19	20	16	5	17	

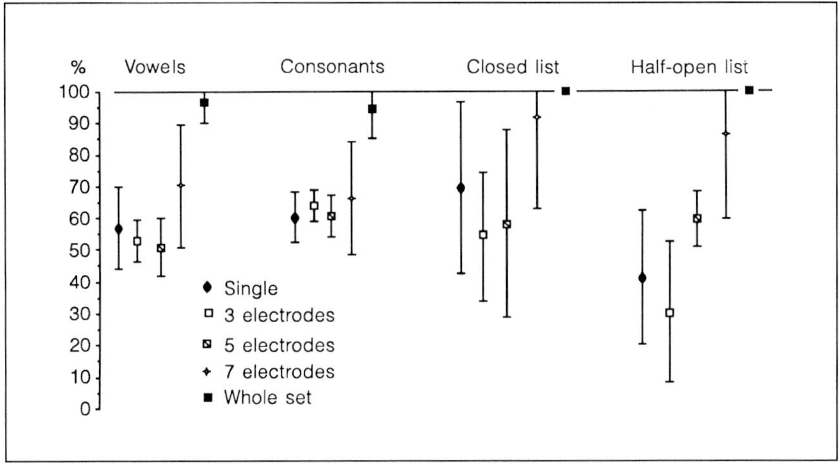

Fig. 1. Mean values of the speech understanding performances with the single-channel system and the multichannel system using successively the 3rd, 5th and 7th last electrodes of the array.

totally ossified cochlea – the coding strategy of this implant is disturbed, and the obtained performances are not better or are inferior to those obtained with the single-channel device. If only 3 electrodes are functional, the difference between the two devices is even more important.

Regarding the 5.4-mm length of the array corresponding to the 7 functional electrodes, one may observe that it is theoretically possible to dig a deeper well in the bony cochlea. But this well is inevitably straight and cannot be curved. Then the proximity of the internal carotid arteria represents a non-negligible risk which cannot be easily avoided at the bottom of this narrow well. Moreover, in a narrow well, despite any adjustments like cements, etc., the array flexibility is a drawback for its insertion and fixation. And, finally, even if 8 or 9 electrodes might be introduced, nothing allows us to be sure preoperatively that they will be all functional, especially because of the bony changes of the cochlea.

On the contrary, the relative rigidity of the single electrode is an advantage for its insertion and spontaneous fixation, which in every case allows full use of the sound signal processing of the implant.

Thus, the Symbion device might easily be used, because each electrode may be introduced separately into its personal bony well. We did not experiment with this device, but we think that a percutaneous plug is an important drawback especially in young children.

The importance of this totally obstructed cochlea must be underlined. Its diagnosis must be performed preoperatively. A simple CT scan enables total ossification to be detected easily. But a total osteofibrous obstruction may have almost normal aspects on the CT scan. Consequently, its assessment may be only a late and disagreeable peroperatory surprise, which can probably be avoided thanks to the recent possibilities given by MRI. The frequency of this total obstruction is discussed. It certainly depends on the ENT specialist's recruitment. Personally, it is more than 10% among 243 implanted patients. However, we think that this frequency will progressively increase in the near future, as its etiology more frequently seems to be meningitis. Thus, it is possible that, owing to the third generation of antibiotics, a lot of people will not die of meningitis, but survive with the handicap of total deafness and totally obstructed cochlea.

Conclusion

For all these reasons we believe that each implanting team must have at his disposal two types of cochlear implant: (1) In about 90% a multichannel device must be used, and personally we use the Cochlear device. (2) In about 10%, when encountering a totally and bilaterally obstructed cochlea, another device must be used. We then use a single-channel system; personally the MXM device.

This opinion became a certainty after we tried to implant a Nucleus device in 2 cases of totally ossified cochlea and, because of the double failure we encountered (making us successfully change the multichannel system with the single-channel device from MXM), finally led to clinical success.

Reference

1 Chouard CH, Genin J, Meyer B, Fugain C, Leveau JM, Dubus P: L'implant cochléaire numérique Monosonic. Ann Oto-Laryngol (Paris) 1990;107:430–437.

Prof. C.H. Chouard, MD, ENT Department, Hôpital St-Antoine,
184, rue du Faubourg St-Antoine, F–75012 Paris (France)

Fraysse B, Deguine O (eds): Cochlear Implants: New Perspectives.
Adv Otorhinolaryngol. Basel, Karger, 1993, vol 48, pp 241–247

Postoperative Speech Perception Results for 92 European Children Using the Nucleus Mini System 22 Cochlear Implant

Josie Reid, Monika Lehnhardt

Cochlear AG, Basel, Switzerland

The approval for implantation of the Nucleus Mini System 22 in children was received in 1990. Since then, 305 European children have been implanted and worldwide, over 1,500 children have been fitted. Preoperatively, in Europe, Australia and the USA, special care is taken to establish that a child does not receive significant benefit from acoustic amplification prior to obtaining a cochlear implant. Postoperatively, the child's progress should be monitored at regular intervals to assess the benefit of the cochlear implant device. One way to monitor the child's progress is to obtain speech perception measures using a battery of tests to assess a hierarchy of auditory skills.

A battery of Speech Perception tests was developed by Cochlear AG and translated into German, French and English. The tests evaluate the benefit of the Nucleus Cochlear Implant for European children between the ages of 2 and 15 years. In this paper we present preliminary results from test evaluations obtained postoperatively.

Method

Subjects

Ninety-two randomly selected children from clinics in Germany, France and England participated in the study. The children were divided into four subgroups based on their age at onset of deafness and the duration of deafness prior to receiving the implant.

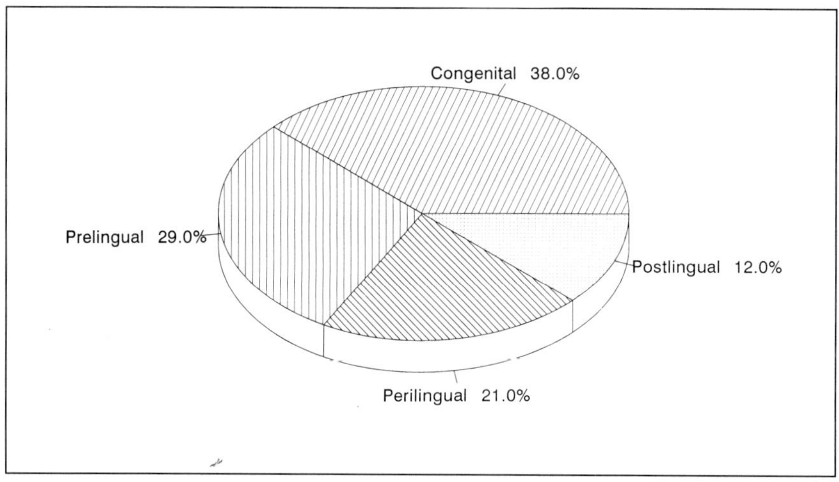

Fig. 1. Language status for children tested (n = 92): congenital (n = 35), prelingual (n = 27), perilingual (n = 19), postlingual (n = 19).

One group consisted of 35 children with congenital deafness, another group consisted of 27 children with prelingual deafness, deafened before the age of 2. The children deafened after the age of 2 were further subdivided into another two groups in relation to duration of deafness. Nineteen children with acquired deafness after the age of 2 were deaf for a period longer than 2 years and classified as having perilingual deafness. Eleven children were deaf for a period shorter than 2 years and classified as having postlingual deafness (fig. 1).

All children received the implant following individual assessment which verified that they received no significant benefit from acoustic amplification preoperatively. That is, the children were not able to demonstrate the perception of spectral information when presented with auditory cues only. Further background information regarding their age at implantation and the experience with the implant is provided in table 1.

The etiology of the hearing loss was attributable to meninigitis for 47% (n = 43) of the children within the study group. Fourteen percent (n = 13) were deaf due to other known causes such as head trauma, anoxia and syndromes. The remaining 39% (n = 36) had no known cause of deafness: unknown etiology was the cause of deafness for the majority of children with congenital deafness.

Speech Perception Measures

Each child's speech perception abilities were evaluated using a range of age-appropriate tests administered via live-voice at normal conversational level (approximating 70 dB SPL) with auditory cues only or with auditory-visual cues. All closed-set tests enabled the child to respond by pointing to a picture. Tests were categorised according to the auditory skill required to perform the task:

Table 1. The range and mean of the characteristic factors for all children in the study group are listed

Factor	Range	Mean
Age at onset of hearing loss	0.0 to 10.4	1.1
Duration of hearing loss prior to implantation	0.4 to 10.4	4.7
Age at implant	2.3 to 13.7	6.2
Age at test	3.4 to 14.9	7.4
Implant experience	2 days to 3.6	1.1

On average the children were deafened very early in life and had a relatively long duration of deafness prior to implantation. These factors are coupled with a mean period of implant experience of only 1 year and 1 month.

Detection of Speech Sounds assesses the child's awareness of speech sounds and is presented with auditory cues only. The Phoneme Detection test contains a range of 18 phonemes presented in combination with several 'no sound' presentations. The child is instructed to respond when tapped on the shoulder by pointing to a 'yes' or 'no' picture card [1].

Speech Pattern Identification assesses the child's ability to differentiate between segmental features using durational and intensity information and is presented with auditory cues only.

In accordance with the child's language level, one of three tests was presented. The tests available were Synthetic Syllable Pattern Discrimination task, Synthetic Syllable Pattern Identification with a choice of four syllabic patterns or Perception of Syllables in Words with a choice of either 4 or 12 words with different syllabic patterns [1].

Speech Identification assesses the child's ability to identify between speech items using spectral information and is presented with auditory cues only. In relation to the child's language level one of two Word Identification tests were presented containing words with similar syllabic patterns in a set of either 4 or 12 items [1]. A third optional test, Sentence Identification, was also available consisting of 6 sentences with similar syntactical structure and syllable number.

Speech Recognition assesses the child's ability to recognise speech related to a particular topic in a modified open-set format and is presented with auditory cues only. One of two Topic-Centered Sentence tests is presented, each containing 10 phrases, composed of simple commands, statements or questions. The child is asked to repeat the phrase. The child's performance is scored as a percentage of total words correctly repeated [2].

Speech Identification with Lipreading assesses the child's ability to identify the word stimulus from a group of three words, two of which are visually homophonous and is presented with auditory visual cues. The Viseme Identification test, which is based on the HAVE test [2], consists of 40 closed-set items. To demonstrate significant benefit from the perception of auditory information in addition to visual information, the child must score above 25 (25/40).

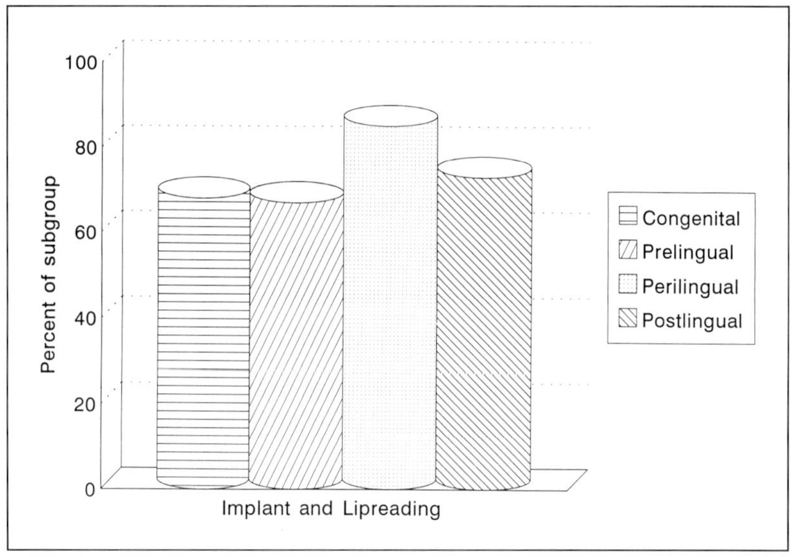

Fig. 2. Postoperative results for Speech Identification presented with auditory and visual cues: A comparison of subgroups revealed no significant differences between their performance. Percentages show children able to score significantly above chance within each subgroup. Total tested (n = 48), congenital (n = 19), prelingual (n = 9), perilingual (n = 13), postlingual (n = 7).

Results

The results reported illustrate the number of children able to perform significantly above chance level for each of the speech perception tasks.

Figure 2 shows the data for 48 children that have been assessed at this stage on the speech identification with lipreading task (Viseme Identification test). The data displays the percentage of children within each subgroup who were able to score significantly above chance. Sixty-eight percent of children with a congenital loss, 67% of children with a prelingual loss, 85% of children with a perilingual loss and 73% of children with a postlingual loss obtained test scores significantly above chance. There was no significant difference between the performance of the subgroups for this task.

The data in figure 3a represents the performance of the total group of 92 children on each of the tasks presented with auditory cues only. All

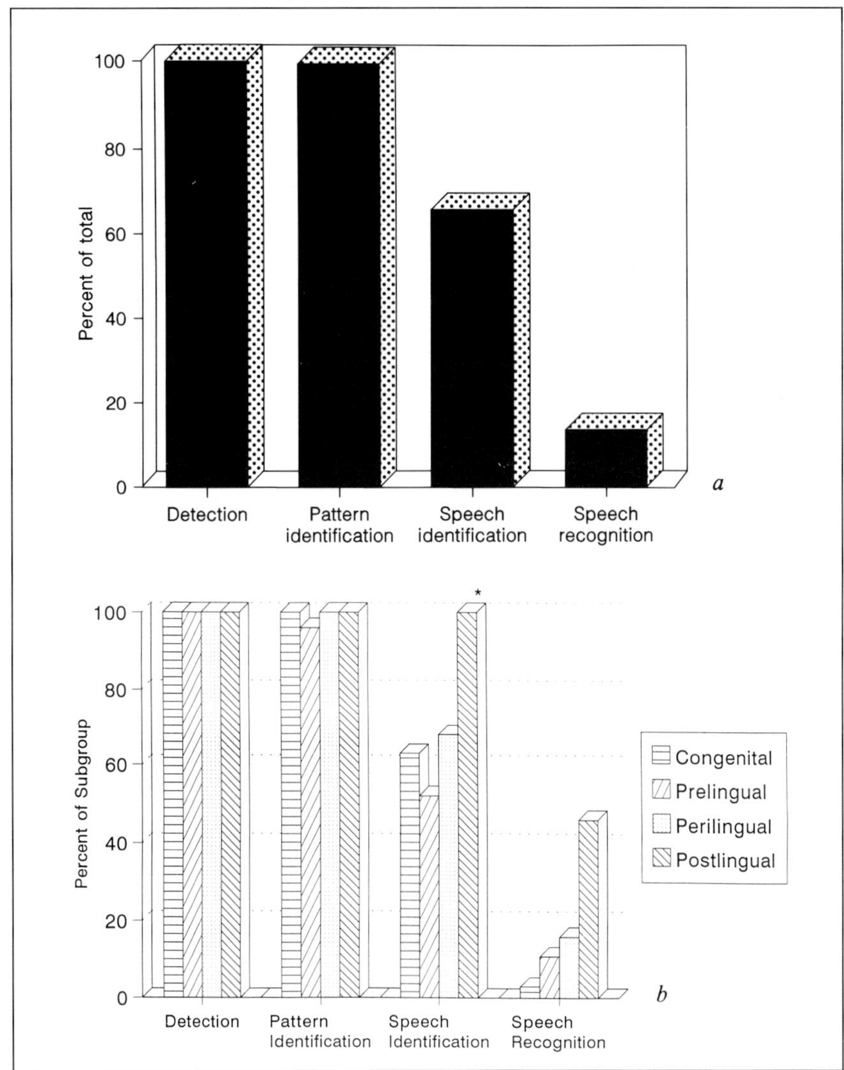

Fig. 3. a Postoperative results for Speech Tests presented with auditory cues only shown as percentages of the total number children who were able to score significantly above chance for each task (n = 92). *b* Postoperative results for Speech Tests presented with auditory cues only shown as a percentage of each subgroup comparing all 92 children. The subgroups consisted of congenital (n = 35), prelingual (n = 27), perilingual (n = 19), postlingual (n = 11). Performance was significantly better for the postlingual children than for other subgroups on the speech identification task. No other significant differences were observed. * $p < 0.05$.

children were able to demonstrate detection of phonemes at a conversational level. With the exception of one child, all children were able to demonstrate perception of suprasegmental features. Sixty-five percent of the test group were able to demonstrate the ability to identify speech in a closed set. Thirteen percent of the children were able to demonstrate the ability to recognise speech in a modified openset format with performances ranging from 8 to 80%.

Figure 3b shows a comparison of the performances for each subgroup for each of the speech perception tasks. A significant difference between the performance of the subgroups was observed for the Speech Identification task only. All children within the postlingual group were able to obtain scores significantly above-chance level for this task which is significantly better than the performance of each of the other three subgroups. However, the majority of the remaining children were also able to perform the task.

Conclusion

Clearly, there are many factors which influence a child's performance on speech perception measures as demonstrated through the diversity in the performance levels for the children within the study group. The test results suggest that children with a later onset of deafness and a shorter period of duration tend to perform better on some tasks than children who experienced the hearing loss early in life and were deafened for a longer period of time. However, the wide range of performance within the subgroups of children suggests features such as onset of hearing loss and duration of hearing loss cannot be used as the sole predictors of the individual's performance potential.

Careful and regular monitoring of a child's performance through repeatable measures such as the speech perception tests described are recommended to confirm the presence of benefit from the implanted device. Ideally, to obtain a true baseline of performance with these speech perception measures for each child, they should be administered preoperatively and postoperatively at various intervals. This would provide more control over the variable of experience with the implant in obtaining comparative data for a large group of children.

Preliminary analysis of the data comparing performance to implant experience, although not reported here, suggests that the trend is for the children's performance on these tests to improve with increasing implant experience. As the mean of implant experience for our study group is only 13 months, we can assume that we are only in the very early stages of realising the full potential of children wearing the Nucleus Mini System 22 Cochlear Implant.

Acknowledgements

Cochlear AG would like to thank all the clinicians involved in the collection of the data for this study from the following clinics listed in alphabetical order: Bradford, Cambridge, CIC Hannover, Kilmarnock, Manchester, Medizinische Hochschule Hannover, Montpellier and Toulouse. A special thank you for their tremendous effort in the data collection to Mr. B. Bertram and to Mr. W. Meyer from CIC Hannover. Also to Mrs. Nadine Cochard from Toulouse and Dr. Thomas Seeger from CAG for their valuable assistance in the development of the French and German versions of the speech tests. Many thanks to Mrs. Sue Roberts for her support in developing the tests and to Dr. Dianne Allum for her advice and guidance.

References

1 Plant G: A diagnostic speech test for severely and profoundly hearing-impaired children. Aust J Audiol 1984;6:1–9.

2 Miyamoto RT, Osberger MJ, Myres MJ, Robbins AJ, Kessler K, Renshaw J, Pope ML: Comparison of sensory aids in deaf children. Ann Otol Rhinol Laryngol 1989; 98:2–7.

Josie Reid, Cochlear AG, Margarethenstrasse 47, CH–4053 Basel (Switzerland)

Different Systems

Fraysse B, Deguine O (eds): Cochlear Implants: New Perspectives.
Adv Otorhinolaryngol. Basel, Karger, 1993, vol 48, pp 248–252

Auditory Brain Stem Implant: Electrical Stimulation of the Human Cochlear Nucleus

F. Portillo, R.A. Nelson, D.E. Brackmann, W.E. Hitselberger, R.V. Shannon, M.D. Waring, J.K. Moore

House Ear Clinic and the House Ear Institute, Los Angeles, Calif., USA

Profound binaural sensorineural hearing loss in an individual who is otherwise physically and psychologically suitable is considered an indication for electrical stimulation. That stimulus can be provided through one of the standard cochlear implants that are available if there is a cochlear nerve to stimulate. However, there is a population of deaf patients without cochlear nerves who are potential candidates for stimulation more centrally. This group includes principally neurofibromatosis-2 patients with bilateral acoustic neuromas.

In 1979, William House and William Hitselberger implanted an NF-2 patient with a single channel electrode at her second tumor removal and she has used central stimulation successfully ever since [1]. From that early start, a large coordinated effort at central stimulation has emerged at the House Ear Institute and now includes a team effort with participating surgeons, electrophysiologists, psychophysicists, audiologists, anatomists and engineers [2].

To date, 25 patients have been implanted with the device which we labeled as the auditory brain stem implant. Of the 25 patients thus far implanted, 18 have devices that stimulate.

Materials and Methods

Patient Selection

The project is an experimental one governed by Food and Drug Administration guidelines. Patients are selected on the basis of total loss of hearing binaurally and the inability to stimulate through the use of a cochlear implant because of the damage to or absence of the cochlear nerves. The patients must be able to tolerate the surgery (which primarily involves the translabyrinthine removal of their acoustic neuroma), and must be able and willing to participate in the necessary postoperative assessments. At this time, they must have English language ability.

Anatomy and Surgery

The translabyrinthine removal of the tumor is chosen because it represents the only approach that provides access to the lateral recess of the fourth vehicle well enough to insert the electrode [3, 4]. The electrode is inserted into the fourth ventricle to sit on the dorsal cochlear nucleus and to provide stability by using the lateral recess as a confining conduit. Location of the cochlear nucleus is provided through anatomic appearance and also by electrical auditory brain stem stimulus using a probe on the brain stem. These electrically derived responses determine the best placement. Other cranial nerves are monitored for unwanted side effects both during EABR and after electrode placement.

The electrode is further stabilized with a tiny piece of adipose tissue directly applied to it at the foramen of the fourth ventricle. Although it appears that the ventral cochlear nucleus would be a better choice tonotopically for stimulation, its position laterally leads to other simultaneous unwanted cranial nerve stimulation.

Equipment

The electrode consists of a 2.5 × 8 mm Dacron mesh carrier which has been found to be well tolerated and stable on the brain stem, and three platinum electrodes attached to the mesh carrier. These are connected to a coiled flexible wire which is brought out through the surgical site to a subcutaneous position on the side of the skull behind the auricle. There it is attached to either a percutaneous pyrolytic carbon pedestal for direct wiring to the external processor, or to a subcutaneous coil for transcutaneous stimulation. The speech processor has been a standard cochlear implant processor configured for single-channel operation. Although three electrodes are currently implanted, they are tested for optimal response and only one electrode is employed for regular wearing. We are presently developing a multichannel electrode array (fig. 1) to improve stimulation selectively and possibly allow use of a multichannel speech processor. Our psychophysics experts have devised speech-processing strategies that have contributed greatly to increased performance even with the single-channel format.

Results

Twenty-five patients have been implanted since 1979 and 18 implants stimulate. Most of the failures were those done in the early years and improved equipment, better placement of the electrodes, and postoperative monitoring of electrode placement have all contributed to that success. One of the earlier failures has been recently revised and is now stimulating. Those patients without troublesome side effects use their implants on a daily a basis and prefer not to be without them. One recent implant patient

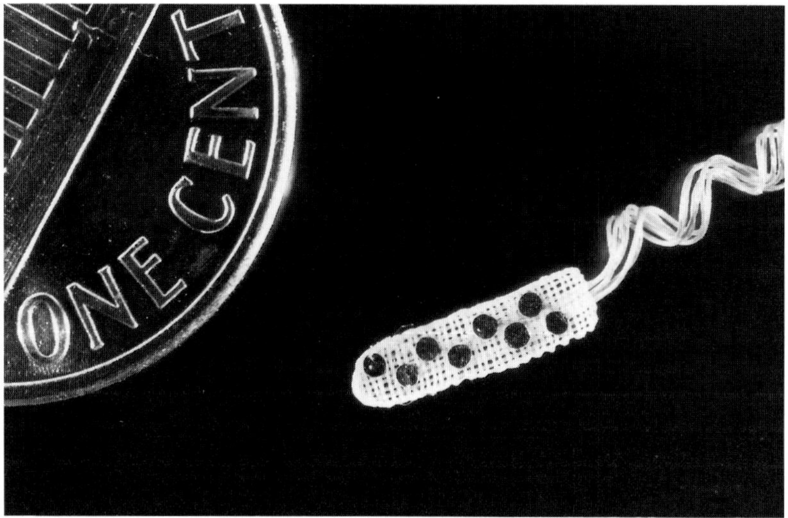

Fig. 1. Multichannel electrode array.

had been deaf for 15 years and has had social adjustment difficulties which have slowed his progress, but he stimulates and he does use his processor, though less than we might desire. All patients can distinguish simple temporal patterns, including number of syllables in a word and stress patterns within the word [5, 6]. All patients increase their speech-reading ability with the implant, some of them dramatically.

Our best patient is able to identify 75% of a 16-consonant set correctly without lipreading and can recognize 15–25% of words in sentences using only the sound through the ABI. He does as well, or better, than our average multichannel cochlear implant patients and much better than most of our single-channel cochlear implant users.

Complications

We have unwanted side effects from cranial nerves VII, IX, X, and XI. Long tract signs have been seen in a limited number of patients. Three patients have experienced what we feel is cerebellar stimulation via the flocculus which sits quite close to the foramen of the fourth ventricle. For the most part, these effects have been avoided by choosing an electrode which provides auditory but no other percepts. There have been no serious side effects dangerous to the patients. Equipment failures have been primarily associated with the percutaneous plugs. These problems have included connecting pin damage and trauma to the plugs from striking the head on overhanging objects, such as door jambs. Revision of the damaged external components has routinely solved these problems.

Conclusion

Brain stem implantation for electrical stimulation of the cochlear nucleus is practical. It provides a viable option for those patients facing deafness from binaural loss of cochlear nerves and in whom a standard cochlear implant would not work. The stimulation derived in some cases has been just short of spectacular and our best subject is able to equal the performance of most multichannel cochlear implant users, even though the ABI is only a single-channel device.

The auditory brain stem implant is a sage, effective, and stable way to provide auditory percepts to totally deaf individuals lacking cochlear nerves.

Acknowledgements

Development of an implantable neural prosthesis requires a multidisciplinary team to work on all aspects of the device. The work reported could not have been accomplished without the entire ABI team. We dedicate this paper to our 25 ABI patients, for their pioneering spirit and persistence.

References

1 Hitselberger W, House W, Edgerton B, Whitaker S: Cochlear nucleus implant. Otolaryngol Head Neck Surg 1984;92:52–54.
2 Eisenberg LS, Maltan AA; Portillo F, Mobley JP, House WF: Electrical stimulation of the auditory brain stem structure in deafened adules. J Rehabil Res Dev 1987;24: 9–22.

3 Edgerton BJ, House WF, Hitselberger W: Hearing by cochlear nucleus stimulation in humans. Ann Otol Rhinol Otolaryngol 1984;91(suppl): 117–124.
4 McElveen J, Hitselberger W, House W, Mobley P, Terr L: Electrical activation of cochlear nucleus in man. Am J Otol 1985;6(suppl):88–91.
5 Shannon RV: Threshold functions for electrical stimulation of the human cochlear nucleus. Hear Res 1989;40:173–178.
6 Shannon RV, Otto SR: Psychophysical measures from electrical stimulation of the human cochlear nucleus. Hear Res 1990;47:159–168.

Franco Portillo, EE, House Ear Institute, 2100 West Third Street,
Los Angeles, CA 90057 (USA)

Fraysse B, Deguine O (eds): Cochlear Implants: New Perspectives.
Adv Otorhinolaryngol. Basel, Karger, 1993, vol 48, pp 253–257

The 8-Channel Cochlear Implant CAP: First Results[1]

C. Zierhofer, P. Pohl, O. Peter, T. Czylok, I. Hochmair-Desoyer, E. Hochmair

Institute for Applied Physics, University of Innsbruck, Austria

There are two fundamental principles for the coding of frequency in the auditory system of normally hearing subjects: the tonotopy (or place) principle and the periodicity principle. Existing auditory prostheses use one or both of these principles in combination. Whereas multichannel pulsatile systems stress tonotopy (i.e. place information) [1], single-channel analog devices have to make up for their inability to provide place information by using more complex stimulation signals [2]. The performance of multichannel analog stimulation systems which are employing several analog channels at the same time is reduced by the presently unavoidable channel interaction which leads to a reduction of the independent information transmitted by each channel [3]. The CAP device suitable for combined analog and pulsatile stimulation is aimed at enhancing the speech recognition by a *constructive* combination of periodicity and place principle.

The motivation for developing the CAP device stems from the results of speech recognition tests with patients using a single-channel analog device. These experiments revealed that speech parameters such as fundamental frequency, signal amplitude, signal duration, the time pattern of the signal envelope, periodicity, and the first formant frequency can be

[1] This work was supported by the Austrian Research Council (grant No. P8347).

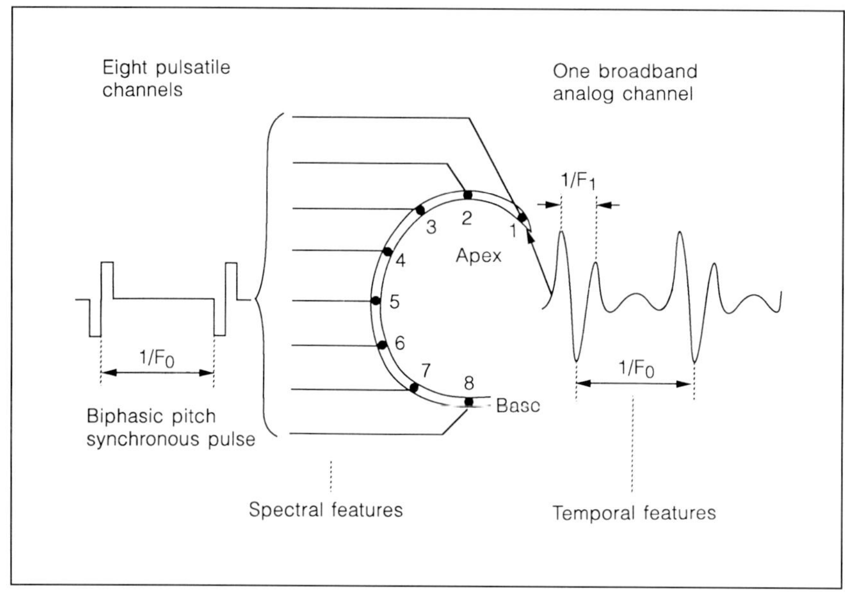

Fig. 1. CAP stimulation strategy.

used by most of the patients. However, the discrimination between vowels with the same first, but different second formant (F2) was limited. The basic idea for the CAP stimulation mode is to complement a broadband analog stimulation channel by simultaneous pulsatile stimulation via additional channels which should convey the F2 information (fig. 1). The stimulation rate of the pulses is equal to the fundamental frequency of the speech signal, the place of stimulation (electrode address) is determined by the spectral location of the F2. It turned out that for optimum vowel recognition, a fixed phase relationship between the analog stimulation signal and the stimulation pulses is necessary. So far, one patient has been implanted with a CAP stimulator.

The CAP implant is suitable for monopolar stimulation with eight electrodes. It contains two independent current sources for the stimulation of the analog and the pulsatile channel. Both current sources can be active simultaneously. The power consumption of the implant typically is within a range of 10–20 mW. The transmission of stimulation power and information is achieved inductively using an rf link [4].

Table 1. Specifications of pulsatile channels

Vowel	F2 Hz	Pulsatile channel address	Pulse delay μs	Pulse amplitude, μA
U	660	2	0	170
O	820	3	900	220
A	1,370	4	0	180
Ö	1,600	5	300	150
Ü	1,870	5	0	180
Ä	2,300	6	0	130
I	2,690	7	0	130
E	2,850	8	900	110

Test Procedure

For vowel identification tasks, the patient had to identify one of eight long German vowels in a 'b' environment (e.g. 'bab'). For each vowel three versions spoken by a female speaker existed. Within one run each vowel was presented five times (resulting in $5 \times 8 = 40$ vowels per run).

For the tests, the most apical electrode (electrode address 1) was used for stimulation of the analog channel. The analog stimulation signal was derived from the compressed and frequency equalized speech signal. The vowels were presented in the most comfortable loudness. The maximum analog stimulation current used was 300 μA.

The electrode addresses for the pulsatile channels were determined by the F2 frequency of each vowel and presented according to table 1. Pulse width was 0.1 ms per phase (biphasic pulses, cathodic first). The delay times between the pulses and the zero-crossing before the dominant maximum of the analog waveform and the pulse amplitudes (table 1) have been determined empirically for best performance. For unvoiced speech segments or silent periods, the pulsatile channels were switched off.

Results

In all, 22 test runs have been performed, 11 with the analog channel alone, and 11 with the combined analog and pulsatile stimulation mode as described above. The results show an average improvement of vowel recognition (% correct) of 15.2%, which is significant at the 1% level (fig. 2). This improvement is clearly due to better F2 recognition (13.9% improvement, also significant at the 1% level).

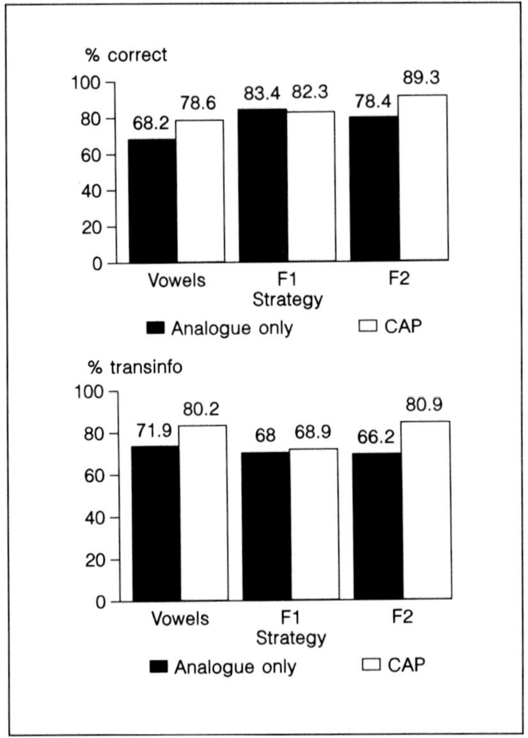

Fig. 2. Vowel recognition test: Comparison of analog only and CAP stimulation mode.

Conclusion

This paper presents the results of vowel recognition tasks of one patient who uses the CAP auditory prosthesis. It is shown that a combined analog and pulsatile stimulation strategy significantly can improve the vowel recognition compared to an analog only stimulation mode. Up to now – at least for the one patient tested so far – the only way to achieve this improvement seems to be to present the pulses synchronously to the analog waveform, i.e. with a rate equal to the pitch frequency and a position within a pitch period near the first dominant maximum (table 1). Other combined analog and pulsatile stimulation modes, e.g. presenting randomly distributed pulses at the corresponding electrode addresses without time correlation to the analog waveform yield an improvement of F2 recognition, but at the same time reduce the F1 recognition so that the overall vowel intelligibility is not enhanced.

References

1 Clark GM, et al: Clinical trial of a multiple-channel cochlear prosthesis. An initial study in four patients with profound total hearing loss. Med J Austr 1983;2:430–433.

2 Hochmair-Desoyer IJ, Hochmair ES, Burian K: The Vienna extra- and intracochlear prosthesis: Speech coding and speech-understanding; in Meyers E (ed): New Dimensions in Otorhinolaryngology. Amsterdam, Elsevier, 1980, vol 1, pp 747–751.

3 Parkin JL, McCandless GA, Youngblood J: Utah design multichannel cochlear implant. Proc Cochlear Implant Symp, Düren, 1987, pp 429–461.

4 Zierhofer CM, Hochmair ES: High-efficiency coupling-insensitive transcutaneous power and data transmission via an inductive link. IEEE Trans Biomed Eng 1990; BME-37:716–722.

C. Zierhofer, PhD, Institute for Applied Physics, University of Innsbruck, Technikerstr. 25, A–6020 Innsbruck (Austria)

Fraysse B, Deguine O (eds): Cochlear Implants: New Perspectives.
Adv Otorhinolaryngol. Basel, Karger, 1993, vol 48, pp 258–260

A New Behind the Ear Wearable Speech Processor for the Vienna Cochlear Prosthesis

K. Burian, O. Klasek

II. Universitäts-HNO-Klinik Wien, Österreich

For the most part electrostimulation offers a great benefit for deaf patients and implants are highly appreciated. Nevertheless, many patients criticize the size of the speech processor which is worn on the body as well as the long cable which connects the processor with the transmitter coil. This was our reason for detecting and developing a miniaturized, behind the ear wearable speech processor (BTE) which has been published last year [1]. In a study on 6 postlingually deafened patients the BTE processor revealed the same or even better performance in the auditory test battery and in the speech tracking compared to the body worn processor. On the base of these results we passed on the prototype of the BTE processor to Mrs. Hochmair and the MED-EL firm, respectively, for further comparative studies on those implanted patients who are under her control in Innsbruck. If our favorable results could also be confirmed we suggested incorporating the BTE processor in the production of the Vienna Cochlear Implant.

Fourteen postlingually, 5 prelingually, and 1 perilingually deafened patients were tested in Innsbruck with the BTE processor (table 1). The results which the patients achieved were evaluated 3–5 weeks after the processor was fitted or for patients in the figures marked with (x) the BTE processors were evaluated immediately upon fitment without allowing the patient to get used to it. With the post- and perilingually deafened patients consonant and vowel identification tests using 16 consonants (96 presentations for each processor) and 8 long German vowels (40 presentations for each processor) and sentence tests (6 lists of 10 sentences each and proces-

Table 1. Results of 20 patients tested with the BTE processor in Innsbruck

Patient No.	Age	Onset of deafness	Electrode location
1	35	postlingually	IC
2	34	postlingually	IC
3	39	postlingually	IC
4	45	postlingually	EC
5	68	postlingually	IC
6	21	perilingually	EC
7	38	postlingually	IC
8	23	postlingually	IC
9	33	postlingually	IC
10	21	postlingually	IC
11	32	postlingually	IC
12	34	postlingually	EC
13	22	prelingually	IC
14	37	prelingually	EC
15	14	prelingually	EC
16	15	prelingually	EC
17	40	prelingually	IC
18	68	postlingually	EC
19	34	postlingually	IC
20	45	postlingually	IC

IC = Intracochlear stimulation; EC = extracochlear stimulation.

sor changed after each list) were performed. The postlingually deafened patients 8–12 have not been tested for their consonant and vowel recognition. The postlingually deafened patients 3, 5, 7, and 18 could not participate in the sentence test. For patient 3, still using an epoxy-coated implant, the BTE processor was at its output power limit and already clipping the stimulation signal.

Figure 1 shows the results in sentence comprehension with the mean values for the BTE processor compared to the body-worn processor. These are 51.5 vs. 46.4% for vowels, 48.6 vs. 39.0% for consonants, and 57.8 vs. 49,1% for sentences. All these tests were significant at the 5% level in the t test.

Additionally, all patients were questioned about the advantages and the disadvantages of the new BTE processor; they all, with one exception, preferred it over the body-worn processor.

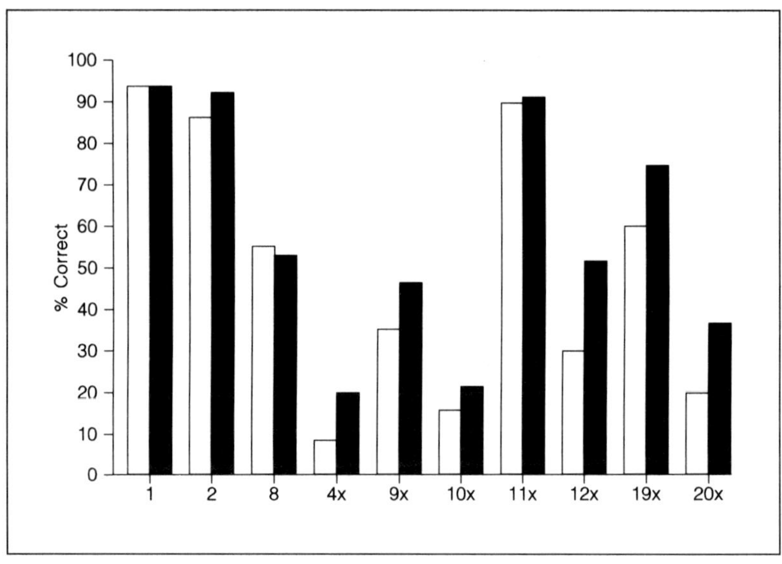

Fig. 1. Sentences, sound only 49.1–57.8%. □ = Body-worn processor at receipt of BTE processor; ■ = BTE processor after 3–5 weeks or at receipt (x).

The BTE processor is now available for all patients provided with a Vienna Cochlear Implant. In view of the above-mentioned advantages almost all patients prefer the BTE processor.

Reference

1 Kürsten R, Klasek O, Szvjatko E, Burian K: First behind the earwearable speech processor for the Vienna cochlear prosthesis. ORL 1991;53:137–139.

Prof. K. Burian, Böhnelstrasse 4, A–2531 Gaaden (Austria)

Fraysse B, Deguine O (eds): Cochlear Implants: New Perspectives.
Adv Otorhinolaryngol. Basel, Karger, 1993, vol 48, pp 261–268

The Laura Cochlear Implant Programmed with the Continuous Interleaved and Phase-Locked Continuous Interleaved Strategies

S. Peeters[a], *F.E. Offeciers*[b, c], *Ph. Joris*[d], *L. Moeneclaey*[c]

[a]Medical Electronics Laboratory, [b]ENT UIA-MISA, and [c]Medical Electronics, Group Experimental ENT, University of Antwerp, Belgium;
[d]Department of Neurophysiology, University of Wisc., Madison, Wisc., USA

Recent experience in the speech-processing strategy for cochlear implants emphasizes the importance of the implementation of both temporal and spectral information in the electrical stimuli delivered to the acoustic nerve fibers.

Wilson [1] and co-workers developed the so-called ‘continuous interleaved’ speech-processing strategy.

Implementation of this strategy in patients implanted with a 6-channel monopolar percutaneous device showed some remarkable results, and seems to be a major step towards a better speech understanding for a greater number of patients. At a time when cochlear implantation in children is becoming a clinical reality, this promises to be very important.

Speech-Decoding Categories

We distinguish two main categories in the speech-decoding strategies: Those based on *feature extraction* and those based on *filtering* of the incoming signal. In the first algorithm (feature extraction) only those electrode pairs corresponding to the localisation of the four maximal spectral peaks of the incoming signal are stimulated with biphasic pulses at the pitch rate (or fundamental frequency) of speech. If no pitch is detected all electrodes are sequentially stimulated with the corresponding intensity. This procedure is mainly based on the *place coding* principle of the ear.

The second category is based on the so-called 'continuous interleaved' algorithm of Wilson's group. This is illustrated in figure 1, which shows the stimulation pattern for eight electrode pairs as a result of stimulation with the word /SO/.

So when we look at one electrode pair, the envelope of one filter output is mirrored by means of biphasic pulses with a total duration of 80 μs and a stimulating frequency of 1.5 kHz in each channel.

This second algorithm was tested in 3 of our patients, performing poorly with the first algorithm based on feature extraction. In accordance with the experience of Wilson and others, all showed significant improvement of performance when stimulated with the continuous interleaved algorithm.

One remaining problem was the poor discrimination between male and female voices, probably due to the poorer perception of the fundamental frequency of speech.

Place Coding

It is widely believed that pitch is determined by the location of the excitation maximum in the cochlea. However, direct recording from single nerve fibers shows that for a given sound frequency, the location of activated fibers changes considerably with sound intensity, whereas the corresponding pitch perception remains nearly constant. Also, according to Honrubia and Ward [2], the maximum the Cochlear microphone can move is by as much as 4 mm towards the base of the cochlea as the intensity of a pure tone increases from 60 to 100 dB. The same is true for the outer hair cells' response. As a consequence, location of the excitation maximum alone cannot constitute an adequate physiological code for pitch.

In other words, the real importance of bipolar stimulation, which gives us the means to stimulate discrete, well-separated parts of the cochlear nerve, is more related to the creation of a real multichannel connection to the brain, than to pitch encoding. For pitch coding, we need more than just place coding. Indeed, we need to control the temperal coding mechanism.

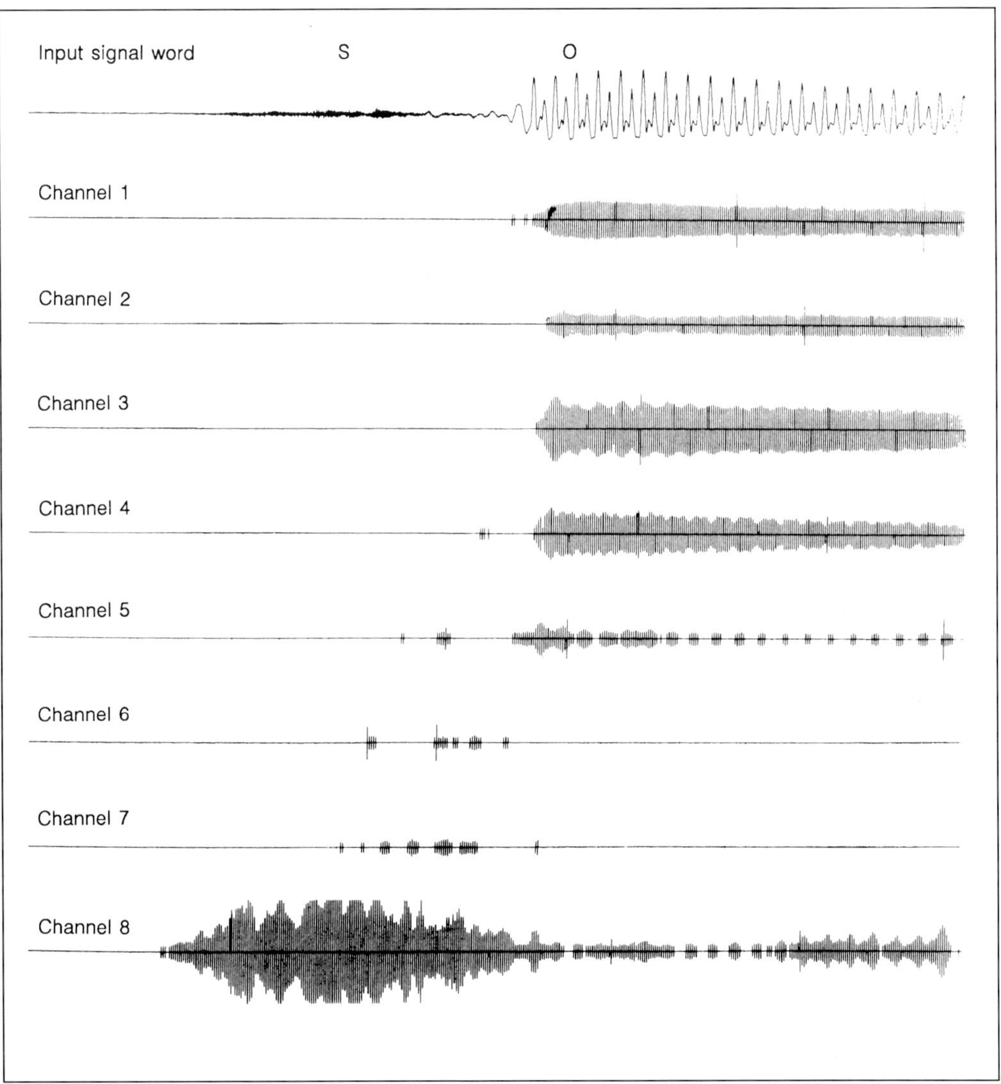

Fig. 1. Representation of the biphasic pulses for the word /SO/. The word SO followed by the stimulation pattern for 8 electrode pairs. Low-frequency channel at the top, high-frequency channel at the bottom.

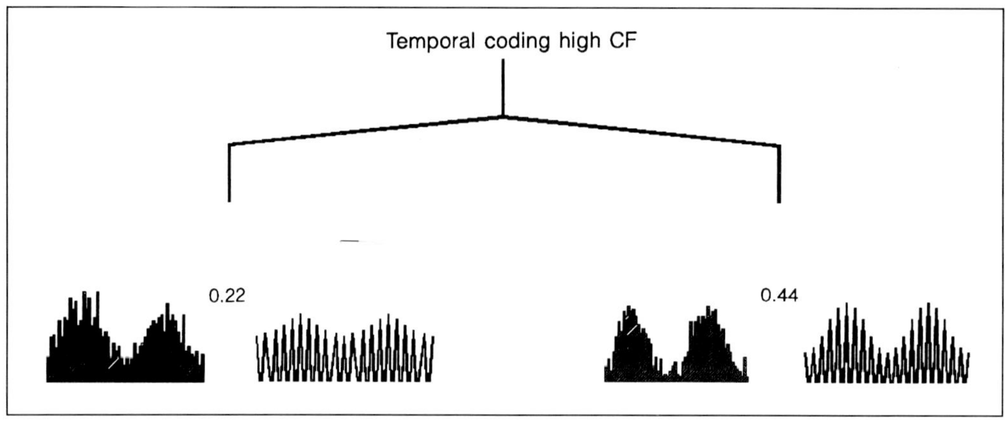

Fig. 2. The periodic histogram for high characteristic frequency (CF) fibers for an AM input signal with a modulation depth index m = 0.22 and m = 0.44. Right from the histogram the rectified input waveform. AM locking for CF < 20 kHz.

Temporal Coding Mechanism

Joris and Yin [3], associated with the ENT lab of Antwerp University and working at Wisconsin University, studied in depth the neural responses to amplitude-modulated (AM) signals. An AM signal can be considered as a simplified formant. The spectrum of the AM signal consists of a carrier frequency Fc with side-band frequencies: one at the carrier frequency plus modulation frequency Fm and one with carrier frequency minus modulation frequency.

Figure 2 shows some results on responses for fibers with high characteristic frequency: (a) the envelope is perfectly reproduced in the periodic histogram; (b) every periodic histogram shows a sharpening of the modulation; (c) when the distance between carrier frequency and modulation frequency increases, the modulation index of the response decreases, and (d) the phase of the envelope is not influenced by modulation depth or by intensity.

Figure 3 shows the responses for nerve fibers with a lower characteristic frequency. We see that: (a) the probability of firing is related to the phase of the carrier (phase locking), and (b) the period histogram shows the modulating waveform.

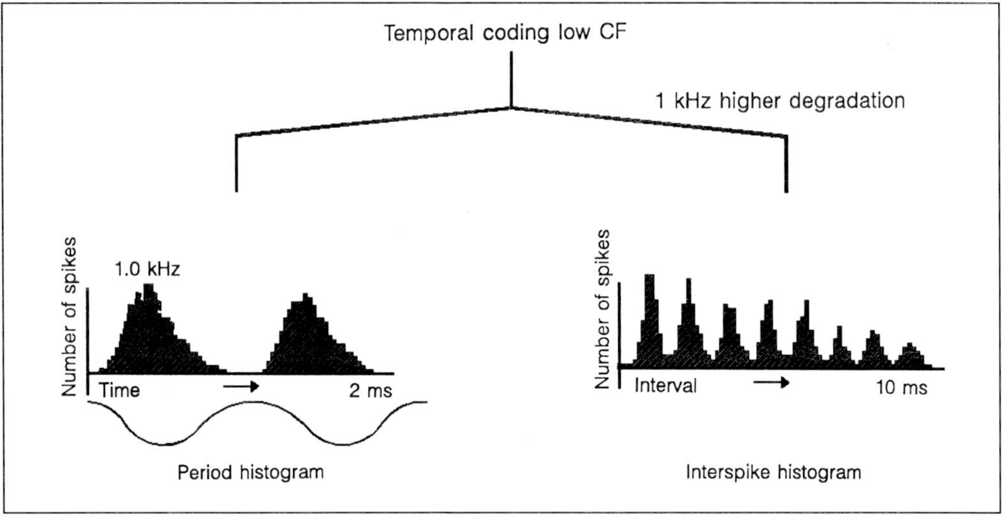

Fig. 3. The period histogram and interspike histogram for low characteristic frequency (CF) fibers. Stimulus is the AM acoustic signal. Phase locking for CF < 1 kHz. Degradation of locking for CF >1 kHz.

Introduction of the 'Phase-Locked Continuous Interleaved' Algorithm

The high flexibility of the Laura prosthesis [4, 5] allowed us to implement those neural response features in a new speech-processing strategy, enriching Wilson's continuous interleaved strategy.

Figure 4 shows the averaged stimulation pattern of one of the higher-frequency channels of the implant. The input signal to the speech processor was a high-frequency carrier (= 3.4 kHz) modulated with a 170-Hz tone with a modulation index of 100%.

The averaged value (lower curve) of the stimulation pattern shows perfectly the envelope of the modulated signal. The modulation depth of the pulse sequences has been enhanced with respect to the incoming signal by means of a nonlinear transformation, conforming the neural activity. For the low-frequency electrodes we introduced phase locking as shown in figure 5. The carrier frequency is 264 Hz while the modulation frequency is 44 Hz. The lower graph shows the averaged phase locking to the carrier frequency, while the envelope follows the AM signal.

4 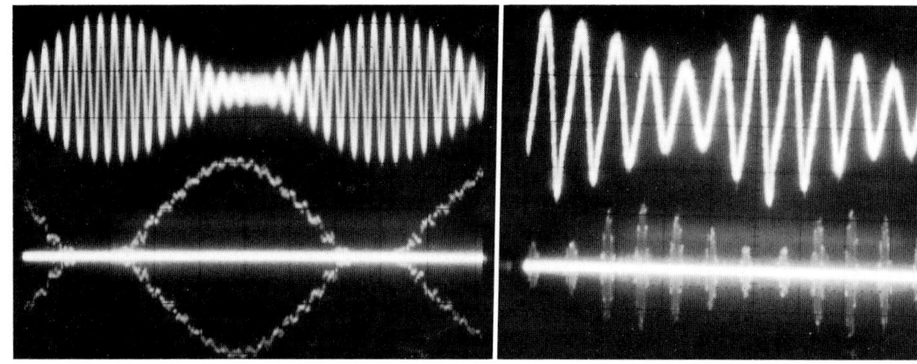 5

Fig. 4. The upper curve shows the AM input signal for the speech processor. Fcarrier = 3.4 kHz; Fmodulation = 170 Hz; modulation index = 100%. The lower part shows the average biphasic pulse amplitude for channel 8.

Fig. 5. Upper curve represents the AM input signal with an Fcarrier at 264 Hz and Fmodulation of 44 Hz, modulation index = 50%. The lower curve shows the average biphasic pulse amplitude for channel 2. For low-frequency channels the stimulating biphasic pulse sequences are phase locked to the carrier frequency.

Figure 6 shows the real time stimulation pattern with this new algorithm in eight channels for the word /SO/. The difference between the first two electrodes and the higher-ranked electrodes is the phase locking.

Recently, we tested this new algorithm on a deaf-blind patient who became deaf 4 years earlier. We first fitted the continuous interleaved algorithm. He scored very well on consonants, but discrimination between male and female voices was poor. The new algorithm immediately resulted in better discrimination between male and female voices. Words sounded more natural. There was improved low pitch perception. Open set recognition of words was amazingly high during the first fitting session with the new algorithm.

Conclusion

If there are enough surviving nerve fibers, we should try to mimic the sound-evoked auditory patterns as closely as possible. This can be done perfectly by controlling the bipolar biphasic pulse patterns along the coch-

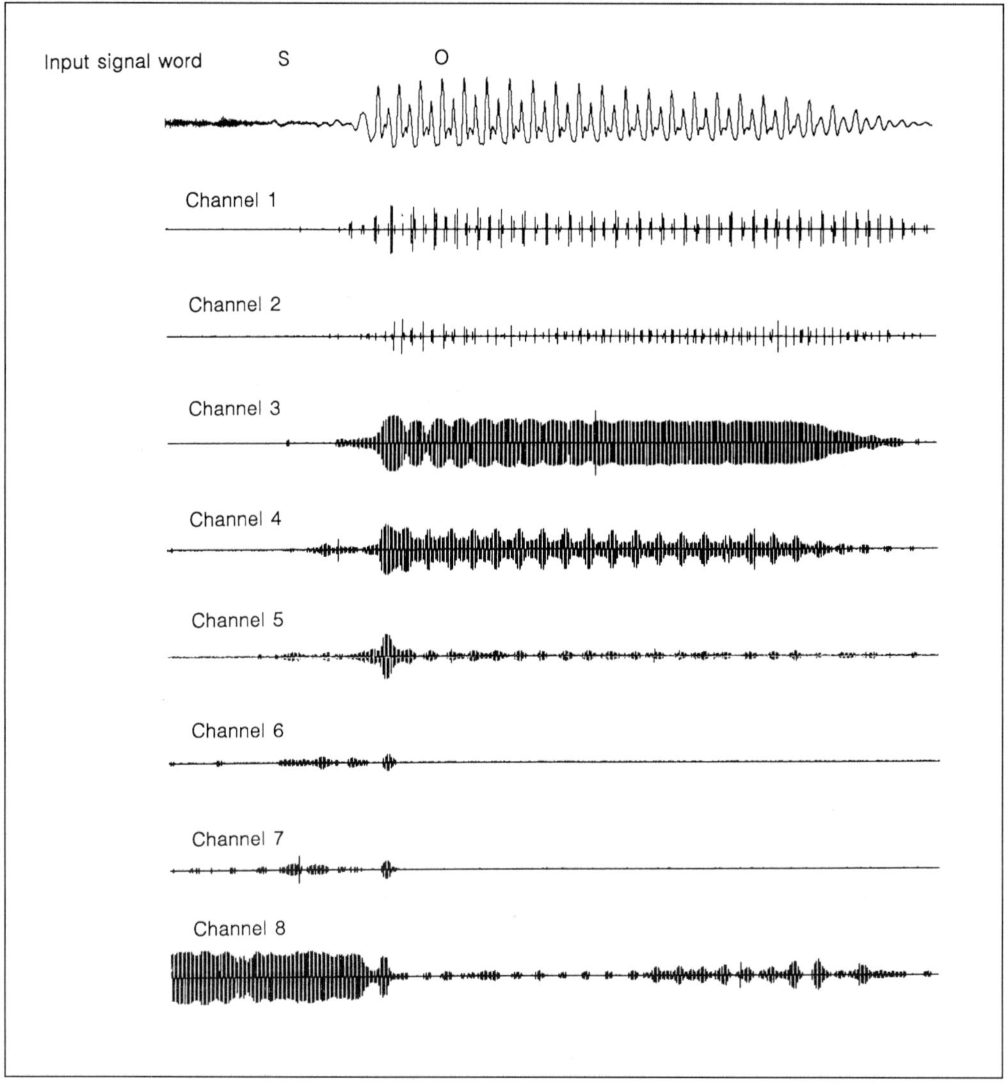

Fig. 6. Biphasic stimulation pattern for the phase-locked continuous interleaved algorithm. The input signal followed by the 8-channel stimulation pattern is shown at the top of the figure.

lea. The brain itself will do the necessary feature extraction when it gets enough information. If nerve fiber survival is very poor, this strategy will not work, and a feature extraction algorithm (some preprocessing) will be more helpful to the patient. The clinical need to adapt the speech-processing strategy to each individual patient is the reason why the new generation of multichannel cochlear implants needs a high degree of software-adaptable flexibility.

References

1 Wilson B: Coding Strategies for MCPr. Am J Otol 1991;12(suppl):1–56.
2 Honrubia V, Ward PH: Longitudinal distribution of the cochlear microphonics inside the cochlear duct. J Acoust Soc Am 1968;44:951–958.
3 Joris Ph, Yin TCT: Response to amplitude-modulated tones in the auditory nerve of the cat. J Acoust Soc Am 1992;91:215–232.
4 Peeters S, Marquet J, Offeciers FE: Cochlear implants: The Laura prosthesis. J Med Eng Technol 1989;13:76–80.
5 Marquet J, Peeters S, Offeciers FE, Van Camp K: La Protesis cochlear 'Laura'. XIV Congr Nac Soc Espanola Patol Cervicofacial, Satander, 1990, pp 155–162.

Dr. S. Peeters, Medical Electronics Laboratory University of Antwerp, B–2000 Antwerp (Belgium)

Fraysse B, Deguine O (eds): Cochlear Implants: New Perspectives.
Adv Otorhinolaryngol. Basel, Karger, 1993, vol 48, pp 269–273

Experience with Four Different Cochlear Implant Systems

Gonzalo Corvera Behar, Jorge Corvera Bernardelli, Antonio Ysunza Romero, Ma Carmen Pamplona

Hospital General Manuel Gea Gonzalez, Mexico City, Mexico

The possibility of the electrode insertion causing greater trauma to the cochlea has always been a major factor in the design of electrode carriers. In 1985, Berlinger et al. [1] mentioned that the risks of neural damage were not clearly known, and, emphasizing the consequences of such damage on children, recommended that cochlear implants in children be limited to extracochlear devices. Other authors [2–5] had also postulated that extracochlear electrodes might be safer than intracochlear.

Based upon these observations, when a children's cochlear implant program was started in 1987 at the Hospital General Dr. Manuel Gea Gonzalez, in Mexico City, the decision was made to utilize extracochlear electrodes.

The present study has two purposes:

(1) Determine the long-term performance of intracochlear vs. extracochlear implants.

(2) Assess our results on congenital and noncongenital prelingually deaf patients to determine our future indications of candidacy with emphasis on the type of implant used.

Material and Methods

All prelingually deaf (congenital and noncongenital) cochlear implant recipients at the Hospital General Dr. Manuel Gea Gonzalez were included in this study. Postlingually deaf children and adults were excluded.

The variables studied were: (a) Number of electrodes used. (b) Position of the electrodes (intra- or extracochlear). (c) The time of use until the appearance of any kind of failure (even if the implant did not fail completely, e.g. one electrode ceased to stimulate). When there was no failure, it was so noted, and the total time of use was taken as the parameter for analysis. (d) The time of use until the patient abandoned our program. This was defined as a failure to continue with formal therapy sessions and/or continuous use of the device, even if the implant was still used sporadically. When there was no abandonment, it was so noted, and the total time of use was taken as the parameter for analysis. (e) The reasons for abandoning the program, if this was the case.

Results

There were 13 patients, with ages ranging from 3 to 29 years (mean = 13.38). Only one patient was noncongenital, he was deafened by kanamycin and/or meningitis at 8 months of age. Thus, the duration of deafness of our population is practically the same as the age (mean = 13.31).

The implants used were: IMPLEX extracochlear, 8 electrode (3 patients); IMPLEX extracochlear, 1 electrode (5 patients); IMPLEX intracochlear, 1 electrode (4 patients); and NUCLEUS intracochlear, 22 electrode (1 patient).

To measure the rate of device/electrode failure, we plotted the number of implants in use without any kind of failure as a percentage of the devices of each type that had been implanted for at least that same number of months. The results in figure 1 show that multielectrode extracochlear implants start failing much earlier than both monoelectrode extracochlear and all intracochlear devices. An analysis of variance shows that extracochlear multielectrode implants failed earlier than extracochlear monoelectrode devices ($p < 0.05$), but there was no significant difference between the latter and the intracochlear devices. Furthermore, even monoelectrode extracochlear implants begin to fail in the long term, but no intracochlear implant has failed in all the time they have been followed-up (only 1 year for the lone NUCLEUS user).

Figure 2 shows the rate of abandonment of the program for the same group. We can see that even in the absence of device failure, at 24 months less than half of our patients who were implanted with a monoelectrode device (extra- or intracochlear) were still routinely using it. The only patient wearing a multichannel device at this length of time was using an extracochlear implant, the other two extracochlear implants had already failed (fig. 1), and the NUCLEUS user has not yet reached this point in time.

1
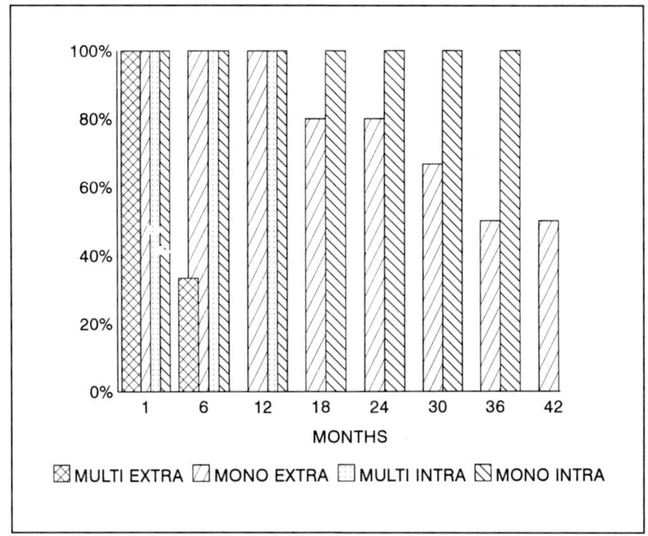

2
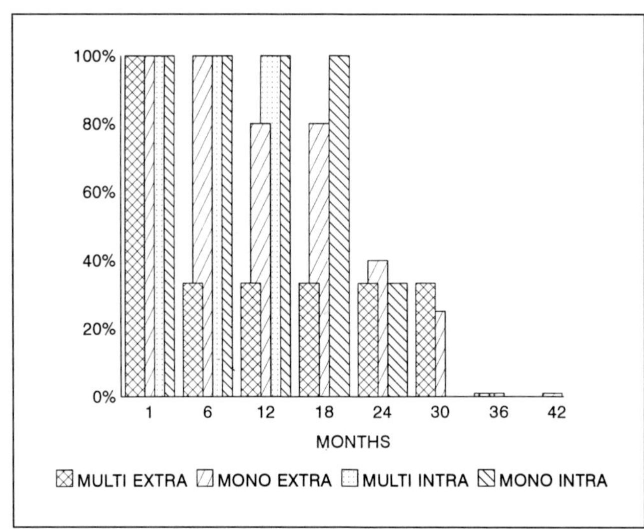

Fig. 1. Number of implants in use without any kind of failure as a percentage of the devices of each type that had been implanted for at least that same number of months. Extracochlear multielectrode implants failed earlier than extracochlear monoelectrode devices ($p < 0.05$).

Fig. 2. Rate of abandonment of the program for each type of device. At 24 months, less than half of those subjects who were implanted with a monoelectrode device (extra- or intracochlear) were still routinely using it.

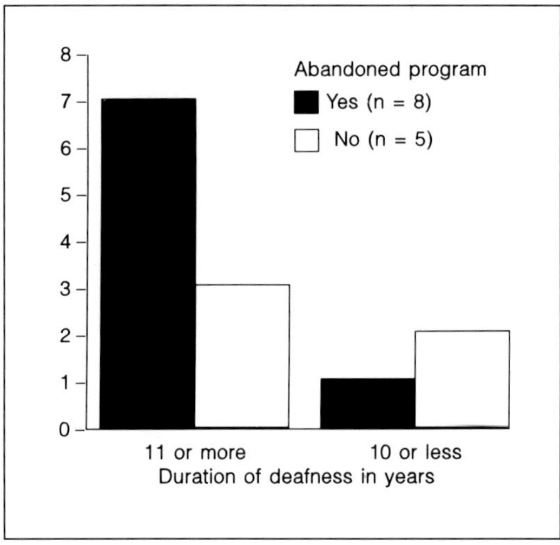

Fig. 3. Prognosis by duration of deafness. Patients who had been implanted after 10 years of age showed a greater risk of leaving the program. The relative risk (RR) of abandoning the program if age was 11 or greater was 2.10. (Greenland, Robins 95% confidence limits: $0.40 < RR < 10.95$.)

As can be seen in figure 3, the patients who had been implanted after 10 years of age showed a greater risk of leaving the program. Seven of the 8 patients who abandoned therapy, expressed dissatisfaction with the gain obtained as the reason for abandoning full-time use.

Conclusion

Our experience with extracochlear implants has made us abandon such devices. It can be argued that better fixation methods could give better results, however, other authors have shown that the trauma caused by intracochlear implantation is negligible [6–8]. We therefore consider intracochlear electrodes those of choice.

The number of electrodes is an important factor to consider. The monoelectrode implants are somewhat less costly, and at-the-ear processors have been developed for these devices; however, our high drop-out rate suggests that even multichannel-monoelectrode implants produce little significant benefit to the congenital and noncongenital prelingually deaf population, specially those implanted later in life. We have yet to determine if multielectrode implants will achieve better results in these patients.

References

1 Berlinger KI, Luxford WM, House WF: Cochlear implants 1981–1985. Am J Otol 1985;6:173–186.
2 Kennedy DW: Multichannel intracochlear electrodes: mechanism of insertion trauma. Laryngoscope 1987;97:442–449.
3 Dillier N, Spillman T: Results and perspectives with extracochlear round window electrodes. Acta Otolar (Stockh) 1984;(suppl 411):221–229.
4 Banfai P, et al: Extracochlear sixteen-channel electrode system. Otolar Clin North Am 1986;19:371–407.
5 Facer GW, et al: Individual data from the 3m/vienna extracochlear implant. Laryngoscope 1986;96:1053–1057.
6 O'Leary MJ, Fayad J, House WF, Linthicum FH Jr: Electrode insertion trauma in cochlear implantation. Ann Otol Rhinol Laryngol 1991;100:695–699.
7 Shepherd RK, Clark GM, Pyman BC, Webb RL: Banded intracochlear electrode array: Evaluation of insertion trauma in human temporal bones. Ann Otol Rhinol Laryngol 1985;94:55–59.
8 O'Reilly BF: Probability of trauma and reliability of placement of a 20 mm long model human scala tympani multielectrode array. Ann Otol Rhinol Laryngol 1981; 90(suppl):11–12.

Dr. G. Corvera Behar, Departamento de Otorrinolaringología, Hospital General Manuel Gea Gonzalez, Calzada de Tlalpan 4800, Mexico 14000, D.F. (Mexico)

Fraysse B, Deguine O (eds): Cochlear Implants: New Perspectives.
Adv Otorhinolaryngol. Basel, Karger, 1993, vol 48, pp 274–276

Cochlear Implants in Europe: Costs and Benefits

Sue Roberts

Cochlear (UK) Ltd., London

Since cochlear implants were first made commercially available in Europe approximately 3,000 deaf European people have been implanted and benefitted from their technology.

The actual price of an implant has probably decreased in real terms because we have not seen the same rise in their prices as we have seen in inflation in many European countries. Relatively speaking they have become cheaper. Nevertheless, it seems that cochlear implants are still quite expensive.

If we look at the price of a multi-channel system it varies between £ 9,000 and £ 15,000. The price of single-channel implant varies between £ 5,000 and £ 7,000. With the limited numbers of patients implanted with each device per year, the increasing regulatory and labelling requirements and the need for commercial companies to financially support research to ensure continued developments in technology, there is never likely to be the significant drop in the price of implants that many have been eluded to or hoped for all these years.

When considering the costs of this procedure we must, of course, add the costs of preoperative evaluation procedures, the surgery, postoperative management procedures, programming the device and rehabilitation programmes. Add to this the cost of repairs and maintenance of the implant system and probably the necessity to replace the external processor at least once every 6 years.

Many cochlear implant centers have been required to budget out all these costs on a per patient basis for reimbursement purposes. The figures will obviously be different for each country but some figures are available.

In the UK for example it is calculated that the costs involved in implantation and management of a child amount to approximately £ 30,000 the first year. In subsequent years maintenance and management visits to the hospital or clinic should cost approximately £ 1,000. Over a 10-year period this would amount to a cost of £ 40,000 per child.

We could assume for the purpose of this exercise that for a postlingual adult the costs would be considerably less, say £ 30,000 over a 10-year period.

There is no doubt when we look at this cost it seems a large amount of money, and it is understandable in the environment of economic recession that we are currently in; it has been quite difficult to convince governments and their social security agencies to pay for this procedure and its associated costs.

Why is it that there has been such a struggle to gain reimbursement for this procedure?

Most professionals now have little difficulty in recommending implantation, even for the young congenitally deafened child.

Most also realise the cost of not implanting a child or an adult, but no one has actually documented them.

For example, what is the average cost of sending a deaf child to a residential school for the deaf rather than providing extra support for the child in a normal-hearing school given that they are able to function more adequately with their cochlear implant?

In the UK it has been suggested that savings of up to £ 10,000 per year per child can be made should they be able to be mainstreamed. Over a ten year period we could therefore save £ 100,000 compared to our cost of £ 40,000 for the implant and management. A long term savings or financial benefit of £ 60,000.

What is the cost to society of a deaf adult who is unable to work because of his deafness versus a rehabilitated adult who is able to return to work?

An unemployed person, for example, may receive an average social security benefit of £ 5,000 per year. Over an average working life of 45 years this would amount to £ 225,000. If they would return to work and could contribute to taxation and the social security system rather than drain from it, their cost to society would be minimised.

There have, in fact, been many cochlear implant patients who have been able to return to work following rehabilitation.

Studies from several years ago in the United States of America suggest that on average the profoundly deaf adult earned only 64% of the income of a normal-hearing person. Assuming that the average yearly income in the UK is around £ 10,000 this would mean that the profoundly deaf adult may earn £ 6,000. If their earning potential were increased by only 20% so that the average wage was £ 8,000 as the result of their implant there would also be an enormous long term saving.

The vocational benefit of cochlear implants is accepted in 23 states in America now where vocational agencies will consider partial or full reimbursement for the procedure based on the knowledge that the individual may be able to return to work.

The figures I have given you may not be exactly accurate but are given to illustrate a point. We should be able, with the help of economists, to provide figures which more than justify the benefits of cochlear implants in monetary terms.

We need to develop the concept of long-term benefit rather than focusing on the short-term cost issues.

There are also many benefits of cochlear implants which cannot be measured in financial terms. For example, how do you measure the benefit of a family being able to communicate with each other in the spoken language the child has learnt through his implant. The pleasure an adult has from listening to the sound of his grandchildren, music and his favourite television program. The pleasure a deaf person has from having their tinnitus alleviated through the electrical stimulation with their implant. These benefits are perhaps immeasurable but nevertheless could be documented by studying the opinions of implant patients and their families on how cochlear implants have changed their lives.

In summary there is to date very little information available in the literature which measures the costs versus the long-term benefits of cochlear implants. We now have a large data base of children and adults whose lives have been changed by this procedure. Hopefully the next few years will see a breakthrough in thoughts and ideas on this subject and some convincing research in the literature which will enable us to ensure that cochlear implants become a largely available treatment of choice for the profoundly hearing impaired individual.

Sue Roberts, Cochlear (UK) Ltd., The Italian Building, Little London, Dockhead, London SE1 2BS (UK)

Subject Index